# PURSUING THE TRIPLE AIM

SEVEN INNOVATORS SHOW THE WAY
TO
BETTER CARE,
BETTER HEALTH,
AND LOWER COSTS

MAUREEN BISOGNANO

CHARLES KENNEY

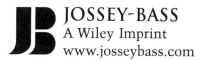

JOSSEY-BASS
A Wiley Imprint
www.josseybass.com

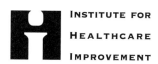

INSTITUTE FOR
HEALTHCARE
IMPROVEMENT

Published by Jossey-Bass
A Wiley Imprint
One Montgomery Street, Suite 1200, San Francisco, CA 94104-4594—www.josseybass.com

*Library of Congress Cataloging-in-Publication Data*

Bisognano, Maureen A.
    Pursuing the triple aim : seven innovators show the way to better care, better health, and lower
costs/Maureen Bisognano, Charles Kenney. – 1st ed.
        p. cm.
    Includes bibliographical references and index.
        ISBN 978-1-118-20572-3 (cloth); 978-1-118-22856-2 (ebk.); 978-1-118-24084-7 (ebk.);
    978-1-118-26570-3 (ebk.)
            1. Medical care–United States–Cost control–Case studies. 2. Medical care–United States–
    Quality control–Case studies. I. Kenney, Charles, 1950- II. Title.
    RA399.A3B49 2012
    362.168'1–dc23                                                                                  2011053063

Printed in the United States of America
FIRST EDITION
*HB Printing*   10 9 8 7 6 5 4 3

# Contents

*To the patients and caregivers working to pursue the Triple Aim and to the amazing caregivers who support us all.*

# Preface

The health care reform debate generates countless areas of dispute yet precious few of agreement. There is, however, a rare and fertile patch of common ground built upon the broad consensus that in the United States today the health care status quo cannot be sustained. Although this notion is well worn, we believe it is also profoundly important, for it leads directly to a foundational question in health care: *Where do we go from here? What will the new health care system look like?* For if the current pathway cannot be sustained, then there must be a new way.

And there is. In fact, this new pathway is hiding in plain sight.

Even with major steps forward, including the Affordable Care Act and the creation of the Center for Medicare and Medicaid Innovation, our national health care debate is too often poisoned by negativity. Yet a quieter, more thoughtful, and vastly more constructive conversation continues among health care innovators throughout the country. This conversation is focused on how to make the system better for patients as well as clinicians, and more affordable for everyone who pays the bills. It is much more than a conversation, of course. It is a formidable movement of innovators whose hallmarks are ideas, vision, *action*. These are people finding a new way; innovators achieving measurable progress on the challenges of quality and cost. The reality on the ground is that the breakthrough work in health care innovation flourishes great distances from Capitol Hill. Solutions to national problems are being designed and implemented at the local level.

We believe these innovators can help show the way to solving some of the toughest health care problems we face as a nation. Their ideas and work, if spread thoughtfully and effectively, can go a very long way to solving much of what plagues our system.

For the past twenty years at the Institute for Healthcare Improvement (IHI) our teams have fanned out across the world, working side by side with thousands of health care innovators. We study, analyze, innovate, and in many cases collaborate on their work from the boardroom to the front lines of care. We harvest, spread, and generate new ideas.

The people and places we write about here have tackled some of the toughest challenges at the heart of the American health care dilemma and done so with a level of achievement that makes them models of innovation. In this book you will learn about innovators who are

- improving quality and lowering costs in primary care by moving care teams out into the workplace;
- applying challenging chronic disease control measures with breakthrough outcomes;
- standardizing excellent care and controlling costs in orthopedic surgery, particularly in the epidemic of total joint replacements;
- leveraging employer buying power to improve quality, reduce waste, and drive down cost;
- paying for care under an innovative contract that compensates for quality rather than quantity;
- finding new ways to care for Medicaid populations while improving quality and reducing cost;
- building a methodical and energetic internal capacity to innovate, to spread innovations and ideas for improvement throughout an organization, and to sustain those improvements at the front lines of care.

These innovations are succeeding now on the local level where they were conceived and nurtured. And although their impact locally has been significant, their potential nationally can be transformative. We do not underestimate the challenges inherent in the large-scale spread of new approaches. Too often health care is slow-footed about spreading emerging best practices. Yet the urgency of the need for improvement coupled with new techniques for effective spread give us a sense of optimism that an emerging trend in health care will be quicker and more certain adaptation of new ideas.

We have seen significant gains in spread in just the past decade. IHI has in fact served as a catalyst for spreading improvements throughout systems and the nation. Proven tools and strategies along with effective partnerships can fuel rapid and sustained spread of the best improvement ideas. We have seen that in many different forms, including our *100,000 Lives* and *5 Million Lives* campaigns.

During his commencement address to the Harvard Medical School class of 2011, surgeon, writer, and researcher Atul Gawande observed that "the places that get the best results are not the most expensive places. Indeed, many are among the least expensive. This means there is hope. . . . We can look to the top performers—the positive deviants—to understand how to provide what society most needs: better care at lower cost. And the pattern seems to be that the places that function most like a system are most successful."

If the innovations we write about here were spread throughout the United States, they would almost certainly improve the quality and safety of health care by an order of magnitude.

In this book we focus on a small number of organizations because we believe these stories reveal a great deal about where our country needs to go. What do these organizations share in common? All are led by men and women of vision—leaders with an obsession for improvement, fearless in their pursuit of better, more affordable care. These organizations and their leaders are imbued with a fundamental understanding of and connection to the transformative power of partnership and teamwork. They are aligned with the idea of integrating health care with public health and social services to get at the full range of health determinants. They embrace integration and coordination of care across organizational silos. They are humble and relentlessly patient centered. All the organizations we write about, with a single exception, are not-for-profits, and nearly all are integrated in either structure or practice. They measure with rigor, know where they stand relative to the best, and spotlight variation within their own organizations in an effort to reduce waste and improve the reliability of care. They aspire to the six aims of the Institute of Medicine's 2001 report—*Crossing the Quality Chasm: A New Health System for the 21st Century*—striving for care that is safe, effective, patient-centered, timely, efficient, and equitable.

But we believe that at the core, what truly binds the organizations we write about together is their pursuit of the IHI Triple Aim:

- Improving the experience of care—providing care that is effective, safe, and reliable—to every patient, every time
- Improving the health of a population, reaching out to communities and organizations, focusing on prevention and wellness, managing chronic conditions, and so forth
- Decreasing per capita costs

Organizations targeting the Triple Aim have gone from looking inward to looking outward, getting outside their walls and reaching out to their communities to improve care overall for populations, whether the population is a panel of diabetic patients or an entire town. And they have gone from paying little if any attention to how money is spent—on tests, procedures, inpatient care, emergency department use, and much more—to recognizing that those dollars are a precious asset for communities, companies, individuals, and our nation. More and more the recognition is growing that pursuing the Triple Aim is not only about a better health care system but also about a sound business strategy and that it is essential to the stability of our national economy.

We want to be clear that no organizations we are aware of have yet achieved the full potential of the Triple Aim—nor, in a relatively short period, would they be expected to have done so. But we write here about organizations that are on the Triple Aim pathway, seriously committed to improving the experience of care and the health of populations and to decreasing costs. And even though none has achieved anything like perfection, all of the organizations we write about have made significant strides.

The Triple Aim is not a new idea although it is a new framework for a growing number of health care organizations. The concept began with IHI's John Whittington, MD, and Thomas Nolan and has evolved over many years. It was first articulated publicly in December 2007 when Donald Berwick, MD, then

CEO of IHI, outlined it during a presentation at the IHI National Forum. In 2008, Berwick, Nolan, and Whittington published an article in *Health Affairs* titled "The Triple Aim: Care, Health, and Cost," in which they defined and made a case for the approach. They noted that improvement efforts until then had been focused somewhat narrowly, and they proposed that organizations view the job of health care with the widest of wide-angle lenses. "Most recent efforts to improve the quality of health care have aimed to reduce defects in the care of patients at a single site of care," they wrote. "Slow progress" is occurring although there is an ongoing struggle "to make highly reliable and safe health care a norm rather than an exception" (p. 760).

The authors had their eyes wide open in recognizing barriers, writing that

> the balanced pursuit of the Triple Aim is not congruent with the current business models of any but a tiny number of U.S. health care organizations. For most, only one, or possibly two, of the dimensions is strategic, but not all three. Thus, we face a paradox with respect to pursuit of the Triple Aim. From the viewpoint of the United States as a whole, it is essential; yet from the viewpoint of individual actors responding to current market forces, pursuing the three aims at once is not in their immediate self-interest [pp. 760–761].

They noted that "rational common interests and rational individual interests are in conflict" (p. 761). And that remains true in many places but it is increasingly less so. In just the handful of years since the article appeared, much has changed in the American health care reform movement. Perhaps as much as or more than anything else, financial pressure, exacerbated by the global recession, has pushed the cost issue to the top of the agenda. This in turn makes the Triple Aim more cogent and timely than ever. One after another, health care organizations throughout the country are deciding it is the right path forward.

Berwick, Nolan, and Whittington also articulated how the Triple Aim might work, noting that a population being managed could be, but need not be, purely geographically defined. "A registry that tracks a defined group of people over time would create a 'population' for the purposes of the Triple Aim," they wrote. "Only when the population is specified does it become, in principle, possible to know about its experiences of care, its health status, and the per capita costs of caring for it" (p. 762).

Essential to successful population management, they wrote, was the presence of an entity that would accept "responsibility for all three components of the Triple Aim for a specified population." This "integrator" role could be played by "a powerful, visionary insurer; a large primary care group in partnership with payers; or even a hospital, with some affiliated physician group, that seeks to be especially attractive to payers" (p. 763).

Success under the Triple Aim would mean thinking differently from the prevailing norm at the time, which was for health care to "respond to the acute needs of individual patients, rather than to anticipate and shape patterns of care for important subgroups." The authors suggest a shift from a focus on sick care to "assigning much more value and many more resources . . . to the monitoring and interception of early signs of deterioration" in a wide variety of conditions (p. 764).

If it is accurate that there is consensus in the United States around the notion that the current pathway is unsustainable, then it comes as affirming news that "pursuit of the Triple Aim threatens the U.S. status quo health system" (p. 767).

In 2007, IHI launched an initiative with fifteen health care organizations that were formally pursuing the Triple Aim (thirteen in the United States and one each in Sweden and England). These organizations committed to applying five design concepts that IHI staff believed would put them on the Triple Aim path: (1) focus on individuals and families, (2) redesign of primary care services and structures, (3) population health management, (4) understanding and changing the drivers of costs to limit or reduce increases across the system, and (5) creating new structures and systems to design and execute changes across entities, cost control platform, and system integration and execution.

After only a few months—by the summer of 2008—the number of groups working on the Triple Aim with IHI climbed from fifteen to more than forty. In recent years the Triple Aim has been the focus of a great deal of our work at IHI. By 2011, we were working with nearly sixty organizations located throughout much of the world on Triple Aim initiatives.

More recently Tom Nolan and others (2010) have made a strong case to pursue the Triple Aim "in a population defined by regional boundaries," according to a recent IHI paper. "Focusing on geographic regions represents a major opportunity to develop new systems of health and health care services that are affordable and sustainable. Regions that succeed in designing high-value health systems will enjoy important advantages—residents of the communities will be healthier and more productive; the communities will be more attractive to new businesses; health care will represent a smaller financial burden on employers, state and local budgets, and individuals." IHI's Triple Aim initiative requires organization-wide commitment along with well-defined parameters and structure. But the Triple Aim is also an idea, a goal, a general framework, and a kind of ideal. It is a fresh per-spective on how to think about health care, and it has captured the imaginations of thousands of stakeholders throughout the country. Some are engaged in the rigor of the initiative itself whereas others are guided by the approach less formally but are in pursuit of the aims nonetheless.

Important thinkers, notably David Kindig, MD, PhD at the University of Wisconsin, have pointed out that the Triple Aim's cutting edge is pushing health care organizations to focus on health and to collaborate with partners in public health and other fields to address the non-medical determinants of health. For those of us working in health care, it is toward this part of the Triple Aim that we have the furthest to go. It will take more than effective improvements in quality and cost to improve health. The innovations at Bellin Health discussed in chapter five and at Kaiser Permanente discussed in chapter seven point to the kind of transformation needed to make a genuine and lasting impact on health.

In the following chapters we relate stories about inspired people doing important work. The innovations in this book are important for their positive impacts in their own communities. Beyond that, they hold promise for helping others find improve-ment pathways forward.

Although the details of these stories are instructive, they tell only part of the story. That is why we also seek here to get inside the heads of these innovators to understand what their thought processes are and have been throughout their improvement work. We seek to understand how they think, how they frame their approach when confronted with difficult challenges. What mental framework did they use to puzzle through problems? What or who influenced and guided their thinking? Have particular theorists, practitioners, writers, or organizations provided a spark or urged them in a new direction? How did they hear the voice of the patients and caregivers, and what changes did these voices prompt? How did they form and execute their new plans? What were the barriers, and how did they think about getting past them? What do they identify as the essential elements of their success? How did they change their organizational cultures and by what means?

Because our ultimate goal here is a practical one—to encourage and inspire others to copy some of this work—we write about what you—as an individual, team, or organization—might need if you wish to emulate work described here. If you are a clinician or administrator and aspire to replicate some of the work, what are the essential ingredients you would need to get started? What are the initial questions you might reflect upon? We make an effort throughout the book to provide clear answers to all of these questions At the end of each chapter we identify components of the work that the innovators themselves believe are essential to their success.

With the spread of the Triple Aim—both the initiative and the idea—we have an increasing sense that it is becoming a sort of true north in health care. For the reality in the United States today is that our country is counting on the health care sector to pursue the Triple Aim and, at some point in the not-too-distant future, to achieve it.

# Acknowledgments

At HealthPartners, we are grateful to Mary Brainerd; Brian Rank, MD; Nancy McClure; Beth Waterman; Beth Averbeck, MD; David Caccamo, MD; George Isham, MD; Rae Ann Williams, MD; Tom Kottke, MD; Art Wineman, MD; and Nico Pronk.

At Intel, we are grateful to Pat McDonald; Richard Taylor; Kevin Carmody; Brian DeVore; Don Fisher, MD; Steve Megli; Wendy Fedderly; Patty Murray; Ian Crisp; Matthew Brownfield; and Mani Shiue. At Tuality Healthcare, we are grateful to Dick Stenson; Janet Meyer, MD; and Amy Sherwood. At Providence Health, we are grateful to Tom Lorish, MD; James Harker; Kristina Herron; Joseph Siemienczuk; Jennifer Bly; Julie Morse; and Mindy Hangsleben. We are grateful to Joan Kapowich, administrator of the Oregon Public Employees' Benefit Board and the Oregon Educators Benefit Board.

At Virginia Mason Medical Center, we are grateful to Gary Kaplan, MD; Robert Mecklenburg, MD; Kathleen Paul; Diane Miller; Andrew Friedman, MD; C. Craig Blackmore, MD; Darlene Corkrum; Sarah Patterson; Kim Pittenger, MD; Charleen Tahibana; and Cathie Furman.

At CareOregon, we are grateful to Dave Ford; David Labby, MD; Rebecca Ramsay; and Debra Read; and also to Rachel Solotaroff, MD, at Central City Concern; and to David Shute, MD, of GreenField Health in Portland. We are grateful to Douglas Eby, MD, of Southcentral Foundation in Anchorage and to the leaders at Multnomah County Health Department in Oregon, including Susan Kirchoff; Amit Shah, MD; and Mindy Stadtlander.

At Blue Cross Blue Shield of Massachusetts, we are grateful to Andrew Dreyfus, Dana Gelb Safran, Deb Devaux, Patrick Gilligan, John Fallon, MD, and Jay McQuaide. We are grateful to former Blue Cross executives Robert Mandel, MD, Peter Meade, and John Schoenbaum. At Mount Auburn Hospital and the Mount Auburn Cambridge Independent Practice Association, we are grateful to Jeanette Clough; Rob Janett, MD; and Barbara Spivak, MD. At Atrius Health, we are grateful to Rick Lopez, MD; Kate Koplan, MD; Les Schwab, MD; and Marci Sindell.

At Bellin Health, we are grateful to George Kerwin, Pete Knox, Randy Van Straten, Jacquelyn Hunt, Amy Seymour, and Patti Eisenreich. We are also grateful to Sarah Novak at Marinette Marine Corporation/Bay Shipbuilding, Fincantieri Marine. At the Orthopaedic Program at Magee-Womens Hospital of the University of Pittsburgh Medical Center (UPMC) and at the broader UPMC system, we are grateful to Tony DiGioia, MD; Gigi Conti Crowley; Leslie Davis; Elizabeth Concordia; Judy Herstine; and Lou Alarcon, MD.

At Kaiser Permanente, we are grateful to Alide Chase; George Halvorson; Marilyn Chow; Lisa Schilling; Jack Cochran, MD; Yan Chow, MD; Louise Liang; Holly Potter; Chris McCarthy; Christi Zuber; Estee Neuwirth; Danielle Cass; Yasmin Staton; Judith Kibler; Teri Whiffen; John August; Diane Waite; Samantha Quattrone; Andrea Buffa; Jennifer Liebermann; Aaron Hardisty; Jed Weissberg, MD; Jan Dorman; Jennifer Lieberman; and Faye Sahai, MD.

We owe a debt as well to a number of men and women at health care organizations throughout the world. We have learned from many health care professions in Jönköping County, Sweden including Göran Henriks, Mats Boestig, MD, and Agneta Jansmyr. In England, we have learned from Helen Bevan, Bernard Crump, and Jim Easton as well as from Derek Feeley, Frances Elliot, Jason Leitch, and Pat O'Connor in Scotland, and Wim Schellekens from the Netherlands. We have learned as well from Uma Kotagal, MD and Lee Carter at Cincinnati Children's Hospital Medical Center; Jim Reinertsen, MD; Jim Conway; Jamie Orlikoff; and Paul Levy.

We are grateful to IHI faculty members Ian Rutter, Catherine Craig, Joanne Lynn, Bruce Bradley, Matt Stiefel, Bonnie Zell, and Trissa Torres.

We are deeply grateful to our friends and colleagues at the Institute for Healthcare Improvement (IHI), including the leaders of the Triple Aim work: Carol Beasley, Karen Boudreau, Martha Rome, Ninon Lewis, Kathryn Brooks, Meghan Hassinger, Kevin Nolan, and others who have invented, innovated, and inspired, including Andrea Kabcenell, Lindsay Martin, and more. We are grateful as well to other IHI colleagues, including Jeff Selberg, Pierre Barker, Penny Carver, Pedro Delgado, Frank Federico, Donald Goldmann, Paul Hamnett, Carol Haraden, Joanne Healy, Amy Hosford-Swan, Andrea Kabcenell, Madge Kaplan, Bob Lloyd, Katharine Luther, Patricia Rutherford, Ken Tebbetts, and Markus Josephson.

A special thanks to Val Weber, Dan Schummers, and Jane Roessner for editorial guidance, expert coaching, and a very special colleagueship.

We owe a debt of gratitude to the IHI board of directors: James M. Anderson, former chairman and CEO of Cincinnati Children's Hospital Medical Center; Michael Dowling, president and CEO, North Shore–Long Island Jewish Health System; Terry Fulmer, dean, Bouvé College of Health Sciences, Northeastern University; A. Blanton Godfrey, dean and professor, College of Textiles, North Carolina State University Raleigh; Jennie Chin Hansen, CEO, American Geriatrics Society; Ruby P. Hearn, senior vice president emerita, The Robert Wood Johnson Foundation; Brent C. James, MD, chief quality officer, executive director, Institute for Healthcare Delivery Research, Intermountain Healthcare; Gary S. Kaplan, MD, chairman, and CEO, Virginia Mason Medical Center; Dennis S. O'Leary, MD, president emeritus, The Joint Commission; Rudolph F. Pierce, Goulston & Storrs, PC; Nancy L. Snyderman, MD, chief medical editor, NBC News, associate professor of otolaryngology, University of Pennsylvania; Robert Waller, MD, president emeritus, Mayo Foundation; Diana Chapman Walsh, president emerita, Wellesley College; and Paul Batalden, MD, a founder of IHI and a continuing visionary.

Our greatest debt, of course, is to the three men who conceived the Triple Aim: Tom Nolan, John Whittington, and Don Berwick. Their vision will change the lives of so many.

# The Authors

**Maureen Bisognano**, president and CEO of the Institute for Healthcare Improvement (IHI), previously served as IHI's executive vice president and chief operating officer for fifteen years. She is a prominent authority on improving health care systems, and her expertise has been recognized by her election as a member of the Institute of Medicine and by her appointment to the Commonwealth Fund's Commission on a High Performance Health System, among other distinctions. Bisognano advises health care leaders around the world, is a frequent speaker at major health care conferences on quality improvement, and is a tireless advocate for change. She is also an instructor of medicine at Harvard Medical School, a research associate in the Brigham and Women's Hospital Division of Social Medicine and Health Inequalities, and serves on the boards of the Commonwealth Fund, the ThedaCare Center for Healthcare Value, and Mayo Clinic Health System-Eau Claire. Prior to joining IHI, she served as CEO of the Massachusetts Respiratory Hospital and senior vice president of the Juran Institute.

**Charles Kenney** is the author of twelve books, including *The Best Practice: How the New Quality Movement Is Transforming Medicine,* which the *New York Times* described as "the first large-scale history of the quality movement." He is also the author of *Transforming Health Care: Virginia Mason Medical Center's Pursuit of the Perfect Patient Experience,* for which he received the 2012 Shingo Research and Professional Publication Award. He has served on the faculty of the Institute for Healthcare Improvement National Forum on Quality Improvement in Health Care.

# HealthPartners

## *Care Model Process and Continuous Healing Relationships*

HealthPartners, based in Bloomington, Minnesota, is the largest consumer-governed, nonprofit health care organization in the United States, employing twelve thousand workers serving 1.3 million people in Minnesota and surrounding states. It is an integrated system, combining a health plan with a medical and dental group that includes eight hundred physicians, four hospitals, and fifty clinics. HealthPartners operates in a state that is home to some of the most innovative health care reform laboratories in the nation, including the Mayo Clinic and Park Nicollet. The overall quality of care in the state is excellent, and costs run about 30 percent below the national average for Medicare patients. HealthPartners costs run even lower—up to 10 percent below the state's average.

In this chapter we focus on HealthPartners' transformative work in primary care, targeted at reliability and the Triple Aim, and we place particular emphasis on the breakthrough work HealthPartners has done on chronic conditions, particularly diabetes.

At IHI, we have worked side-by-side with HealthPartners on a variety of initiatives for more than a decade. We believe it is one of the great health care organizations anywhere in the world. In its pursuit of the Triple Aim, HealthPartners has built a care delivery system based on a rock-solid foundation of *reliability, customization, access,* and *coordination* of care. A conservative estimate suggests that spreading HealthPartners' best practices throughout the nation has the potential to save *$2 trillion over the next decade.*

## Hearing a Call to Change the System

In the life of a major, integrated health care system, it is often difficult to identify the critical moment, *the* event, that will serve as a kind of true north for at least a decade going forward. But Dr. Brian Rank can pinpoint that moment for HealthPartners. It came in 2001 with the publication of *Crossing the Quality Chasm: A New Health System for the 21st Century,* a report by the Institute of Medicine (IOM). This report captivated Rank like few other books, reports, or papers he had ever read.

"The *Chasm* report was the turning point for us," says Rank, a medical oncologist who serves as medical director for HealthPartners Medical Group & Clinics. "It really does set out a road map for moving from visit-based care to continuous healing relationships. It speaks directly to chronic disease management. It's both a theoretical and practical appeal to the issues that continue to plague American health care and health care in the world in general."

When *Crossing the Quality Chasm* was published, Rank was in his third year as director of the HealthPartners medical group. He had completed his training at the University of Minnesota in 1985, "when quality in health care was, *'Go do a good job and don't harm anybody.'*" But in the ensuing years he and his colleagues on the HealthPartners leadership team had seen disconnections throughout health care—an obvious lack of coherence; an absence of intelligent processes to make things fit together for patients. Like many physicians searching for a better way forward, he had been struck by the earlier IOM report *To Err Is Human* (Kohn, Corrigan, & Donaldson, 2000).

"*To Err Is Human* hit on the American psyche," says Rank. "It was all over the media—100,000 preventable deaths in hospitals every year. Safety experts were on TV saying 'don't go into the hospital without a friend so no one does anything bad to you.'" But to Rank and his associates at HealthPartners, the *Chasm* report—which received a fraction of the public attention heaped upon *To Err Is Human*—was a vastly more important document, for it spoke to the absence of a *system* to provide better, safer, more efficient and affordable care. In other words, it went directly toward what Rank and his colleagues wanted to accomplish at HealthPartners. The *Chasm* report noted that although *To Err Is Human* "was a call for action to make care safer, this report is a call for action to improve the American health care delivery system as a whole, in all its quality dimensions, for all Americans" (p. 2).

The very idea embodied in the opening of the report— that health care "routinely fails to deliver its potential benefits" (p. 1)—was a damning indictment of the world's most scientifically advanced society.

"The current care systems cannot do the job," stated the report. "Trying harder will not work. Changing systems of care will" (p. 4). The report stated that

> health care has safety and quality problems because it relies on outmoded systems of work. Poor designs set the workforce up to fail, regardless of how hard they try. If we want safer, higher-quality care, we will need to have redesigned systems of care, including the use of information technology to support clinical and administrative processes [p. 4].

> Americans should be able to count on receiving care that meets their needs and is based on the best scientific knowledge. Yet there is strong evidence that this frequently is not the case [p. 1].

Although the *Chasm* report was all but ignored at many if not most organizations throughout the nation, it was immediately embraced at HealthPartners, where CEO Mary Brainerd and her leadership team were united in their belief that this report carried seminal importance. "It was such a powerful description of the things that were standing in the way of delivering the care that everyone who goes into health care intends to deliver," says

Brainerd. "It was a really clear articulation of the things we need to overcome in order to get there."

## Recognizing a Broken System—A *Nonsystem*

The report was also an affirmation of what Brainerd, Rank, and their colleagues had believed for some time—that the health care system was badly broken; in fact, that it was not a system at all. Rank and his administrative counterpart Nancy McClure, senior vice president of HealthPartners Medical Group & Clinics, read the report as soon as it was published, and McClure recalls it as a "seismic shift" in health care. The report defined the quality goal for American health care as embodied within six aims—it is care that is "safe, effective, patient centered, timely, efficient, and equitable" (p. xi).

"We knew the minute we read it—the *nanosecond* we read it— that the six aims would give us a framework going forward," says McClure. "We knew the chassis was broken. Health care had not developed reliable processes and systems like other industries."

The old system—or more precisely nonsystem—was built on a platform of presumed physician omniscience, the idea that a doctor, well-trained in medical school, working essentially alone in a solo practice or independently in a group practice, would know what was best for every patient. Although that approach served many patients very well, indeed, it also meant that best practices were not updated and applied consistently. It meant enormous unneeded variation in care, not only from one area of the country to another but also among clinics and doctors in the same organization. "You are assuming, without a system, that every doctor is going to remember what to do and just do the right thing," says McClure. "It creates chaos."

That lack of a system, says Brian Rank, essentially told doctors that "*if you just try harder you can get better.* Every clinician that I know is already working as hard as they can." Prior to *Crossing the Quality Chasm*, Rank says, doctors would conduct a variety of improvement projects that would seem, at the moment, quite successful. But "when we turned our attention away, whatever it [was] we improved went back to whatever it was before, because the system didn't change."

"Because," McClure interjects, "*there was no system.*"

Brainerd, Rank, McClure, and others saw the report both as an indictment of what was wrong with health care and as the beginning of a road map for what needed to change. They were drawn to the six aims as a way to define quality and measure improvement. "It was the first time that anyone had articulated a set of dimensions where efficiency, effectiveness, safety, and patient centeredness were all considered elements of quality," says McClure. "Before that, technical quality was typically seen as in opposition to utilization management—as if you couldn't be efficient and have high quality at the same time." Table 1.1 displays a comparison that Rank believes tells much of the *Chasm* story.

### Table 1.1. Simple Rules for the Twenty-First-Century Health Care System

| Current Approach | New Rule |
|---|---|
| Care is based primarily on visits. | Care is based on continuous healing relationships. |
| Professional autonomy drives variability. | Care is customized according to patient needs and values. |
| Professionals control care. | The patient is the source of control. |
| Information is a record. | Knowledge is shared and information flows freely. |
| Decision making is based on training and experience. | Decision making is evidence based. |
| Do no harm is an individual responsibility. | Safety is a system property. |
| Secrecy is necessary. | Transparency is necessary. |
| The system reacts to needs. | Needs are anticipated. |
| Cost reduction is sought. | Waste is continuously decreased. |
| Preference is given to professional roles over the system. | Cooperation among clinicians is a priority. |

*Source:* Kohn, Corrigan, & Donaldson, 2000, Table 3-1.

In 2001, HealthPartners publicly incorporated the six aims of *Chasm* into its mission, vision, and organizational goals and Brainerd changed the annual planning process so that goals and plans had to relate to the six aims.

## Focusing on Reliability and Standardization

Rank, McClure, and others at HealthPartners convened physician and administrative teams from the medical group to focus on creating reliable systems of care that could be implemented across the HealthPartners organization. They were asking the doctors to think beyond a particular visit or individual and more toward how the clinical teams could collaborate for the patient's benefit; how they could reduce variation and achieve a higher degree of standardization around agreed-upon best practices.

Thinking differently is often a challenge in health care, but it was nothing new at HealthPartners. There was something iconoclastic in the organization's DNA and certainly in its history. As a member-owned and member-governed cooperative, its governance structure has helped to make it particularly patient focused. When patients control the board—when patients *are* the board—it makes a difference.

"We have a history of saying we are not just here to do business as usual," says Brainerd. The organization was seen as somewhat revolutionary when it was started back in the 1950s, with its intensive consumer focus. Located on Como Avenue, it was nicknamed "Commies on Como" early on and Brainerd says that the intent was never to be a traditional health system. "Consumers hiring doctors to work on a salary in a clinic instead of in a small business was revolutionary," she says. HealthPartners was posting quality outcomes on the Web for consumers to use as early as 1997, and Brainerd points to this practice as evidence of the organization's new approach. "People began with an idea that this was a different model, a different set of values, and I think we have done a pretty good job over time in living those out," she says. "I think the recent work is bigger scale. We are a bigger system. The challenges are greater."

## Zen and the Art of Physician Autonomy

As Brainerd, Rank, and the leadership team worked to create a new system of care, an article by Dr. James Reinertsen (2003) was published that captured their attention. Dr. Reinertsen had formerly practiced at Park Nicollet, a Twin Cities neighbor to HealthPartners. He had since moved on to become CEO of Beth Israel Deaconess Medical Center, a Harvard teaching hospital in Boston. The article, published in 2003 in *Annals of Internal Medicine*, was titled "Zen and the Art of Physician Autonomy Maintenance," and Rank regarded it as a superb description of a major flaw in American health care: the failure to standardize knowledge and to apply it broadly and consistently for the benefit of patients. "For me, it was a seminal article," says Rank. "It takes on the myth that every doctor has to figure out the science for everything all the time. In oncology, we have national cooperative trials where the standard of care is specified. But for a lot of medicine—look at the Dartmouth Atlas—there is wide variation."

Many physicians, says Rank, apply the knowledge and techniques they acquired as medical students twenty or more years ago even in cases where new techniques have proven superior. Rank knew this from experience of course, but the Reinertsen article powerfully reinforced that notion. "Every doctor, even today, is trained in a medical training system in which we all re-create wheels," says Rank. "You never trust anyone to synthesize that science, and you are supposed to understand and have read all seventeen thousand randomized clinical trials this year added on to what you knew for last year and then synthesize the science yourself. That is a total impossibility and it is a massive failure pathway."

The article "also says that the systems that we work in can make us either better doctors or worse doctors," Rank continues. "If we have seven different preps for carpal tunnel surgery, chances are you are going to get the wrong one much of the time. . . . [Reinertsen's] epiphany around recreating wheels and practicing alone together was highly poignant for me and it also allowed us to enfold physician behavior into the scaffolding [for our system] in ways that value their training, their experience, and don't ask them to recreate wheels all the time."

Rank's comments echo the words of Dr. Atul Gawande in his commencement address to the 2011 class at the Harvard Medical School. Gawande told the graduates that "the core structure of medicine—how health care is organized and practiced—emerged in an era when doctors could hold all the key information patients needed in their heads and manage everything required them-selves. . . . We were craftsmen. We could set the fracture, spin the blood, plate the cultures, administer the antiserum. The nature of the knowledge lent itself to prizing autonomy, inde-pendence, and self-sufficiency among our highest values, and to designing medicine accordingly. But you can't hold all the information in your head any longer, and you can't master all the skills."

In his article Reinertsen also observed that although physi-cians placed extraordinary value on their autonomy, marketplace forces were pushing them to "practice evidence-based medi-cine i.e. to make effective use of the very science on which we base our profession."

In addition to *Crossing the Quality Chasm* and "Zen and the Art of Physician Autonomy Maintenance," another source of ideas that influenced the HealthPartners' leadership team was Dr. Donald Berwick's 1999 IHI Forum keynote address, called "Escape Fire." Brainerd was inspired by what she called Berwick's "emotionally compelling call to action. His message was that we cannot any longer afford to do things in a haphazard way. We can't trust only the individual. We need to create teams and standards and expec-tations of ourselves that are different than anything we have ever done before. We need to institute rigor around process change and do that together with a goal of creating something that doesn't exist anywhere."

It was a message very much consistent with the themes struck in *Chasm* and Reinertsen's article. Around the same time, Tom Nolan, a statistician and IHI Senior Fellow, attended a HealthPartners board retreat. Nolan had worked with the HealthPartners team for some time, and he had emerged as one of the leading thinkers in the health care improvement universe. Nolan "really pushed our board to set more ambitious goals," says Rank. "We had a very serious discussion about how to create that balance between what is aspirational and maybe imaginary and what is real but maybe not very much of a transformational step. I think we came out of that with greater clarity of how hard we wanted to push ourselves."

## Pursuing Perfection: A New and Better System of Care?

At that point the question for Brainerd, Rank, and the leadership team was how to translate their vision and aspirations into reality. "We were looking to make big-scale changes and had no clue about how to do that," says Brainerd. Then they heard some serendipitous news. Not long after publication of the *Chasm* report, and just as HealthPartners was looking for guidance in 2001, IHI announced its Pursuing Perfection program, intended to help health care organizations "make dramatic improvements in performance across the organization, resulting in a considerably more efficient and effective health care system." In all, seven organizations in the United States, including HealthPartners, and six in Europe were selected for Pursuing Perfection (from among several hundred applicants). Working with faculty from IHI as well as from other organizations (including, for example, Hackensack University Medical Center and Cincinnati Children's Hospital Medical Center), HealthPartners began rethinking its care delivery process.

A major challenge that stood stubbornly in HealthPartners' path was an inability to spread good work throughout the organization. "We could do projects, but we couldn't spread improvements very capably," says Brainerd. "We could do one really cool thing in three clinics and then we would develop a toolkit to share with the seventeen other clinics, but that approach was not effective. It was frustrating, and we couldn't figure out exactly what was standing in the way." This troubled Brainerd. She wanted to do something different and dramatic to convey as vividly as she could to her employees what was needed to make fundamental change within the organization. After internal discussions she did something highly unusual: she commissioned playwright Syl Jones to write an original stage play as a way to help capture the attention of HealthPartners employees and to generate discussion about changes needed in the care process.

*Fire in the Bones* was designed to raise awareness among employees "of the dramatic transformation that our organization is undertaking to deliver care that is measurably safer, more timely, effective, efficient, equitable and patient-centered," wrote Brainerd in a message to employees. The story focuses on the response of friends to the death of a middle-aged social worker. Questions are raised about whether, if care had been delivered differently, she might still be alive. Essential aspects of the performance called into question the approach to work at HealthPartners. As a result, seeing the play was a powerful emotional experience— and not a particularly pleasant one—for many who worked at HealthPartners.

Every HealthPartners doctor and staff member was provided an opportunity to travel to a theater to see the production performed by a company of professional actors. After a performance was completed, employees in the audience engaged in a discussion with Brainerd and other senior leaders. These were sometimes tense, difficult discussions. Staff members were upset or even angry that their care delivery was portrayed as less than excellent in the play. This was, of course, by design. The play "dramatizes some of the very real flaws in our current systems," Brainerd wrote to the staff, "but most importantly it provides an inspirational depiction of how different health care could be."

At the start of the Pursuing Perfection program, leaders at IHI and the Robert Wood Johnson Foundation, which funded the program for the U.S. sites, urged participants to follow a 2-5-all formula: that is, to improve their process in two areas, then in five areas, and then spread the new process throughout the organization. Brainerd and colleagues were uncomfortable with that approach and said so, but they were convinced to follow the path nonetheless. Just a year into it, however, it was not working for them.

"We were concerned with improving care one condition at a time," says McClure. "If we focus on diabetes, then asthma, then depression, and so forth, we tend to add costs and complexity to the system. We needed to create a chassis that could produce reliable results across multiple conditions and we weren't going to do that if we focused on one condition at a time. Patients don't actually come in that way anyway." Thus HealthPartners embarked on a midcourse correction "to design a reliable system in which we can produce results across multiple conditions and not do it one condition at a time."

Beth Waterman, a registered nurse and HealthPartners' chief improvement officer, who was then vice president of primary care and clinic operations and project director for Pursuing Perfection, reflected the leadership team's frustration when she said that the clinicians were working very hard but were not getting better results. Waterman and other leaders were not at all comfortable with the reactive, visit-focused model of care and wanted something better, but they weren't sure what that was exactly.

The Pursuing Perfection experience revealed some flaws at HealthPartners, notably the organization's ongoing struggle to become more patient centered. In engaging with other program participants, the HealthPartners team saw an approach to patient centeredness far beyond anything they had done. Cincinnati Children's Hospital Medical Center, for example, had embraced the idea of including patients and their families in virtually everything the hospital did. This reached the point where Lee Carter, the Cincinnati Children's Hospital board chair, insisted that parents be present at every board meeting. Carter said there was nothing like the power of a parent looking him in the eye and telling him that the hospital had hurt that parent's child to accelerate the hospital's effort at safety and quality improvement. Cincinnati Children's Hospital also has parents serving on both its board and its Patient Care Committee.

When the HealthPartners team saw this sort of patient engagement, "we really took it to heart," says Waterman. "We saw that we should be doing a lot better." The team adopted the Cincinnati Children's concept, made sure to include patients in care design sessions, and created several patient advisory councils.

## Rewiring the Whole Thing: The Wagner Model

But how would they provide reliable care to every patient every time? How could they tackle "in-between visit care"? How could they reach out to patients—many of them chronically ill—and get them in for the treatments and tests they most needed? Mary Brainerd had said they needed to "rewire the whole thing"; to build a system capable of providing reliable, standardized care to every patient every time.

Around this time Dr. Edward H. Wagner, of Group Health in Seattle, visited HealthPartners. Since 1998, Wagner and his colleagues had been developing and disseminating Wagner's *chronic care model* at the Group Health Research Institute and the MacColl Center for Health Care Innovation (Figure 1.1).

The model combines evidenced-based medicine and clinical teamwork to provide care for patients with chronic conditions, and there had been some discussion about whether this model might work within HealthPartners. The Web site for the Group Health Research Institute's program Improving Chronic Illness Care (1998) identifies the essential elements of a health care system that delivers high-quality chronic disease care under the chronic care model. These elements are the community, the health system, self-management support, delivery system design, decision support, and clinical information systems. Evidence-based change concepts related to each element can be used to

## Figure 1.1. Wagner's Chronic Care Model

Community
Resources and Policies

Health Systems
Organization of Health Care

Self-Management Support

Delivery System Design

Decision Support

Clinical Information Systems

Informed, Activated Patient

Productive Interactions

Prepared, Proactive Practice Team

**Improved Outcomes**

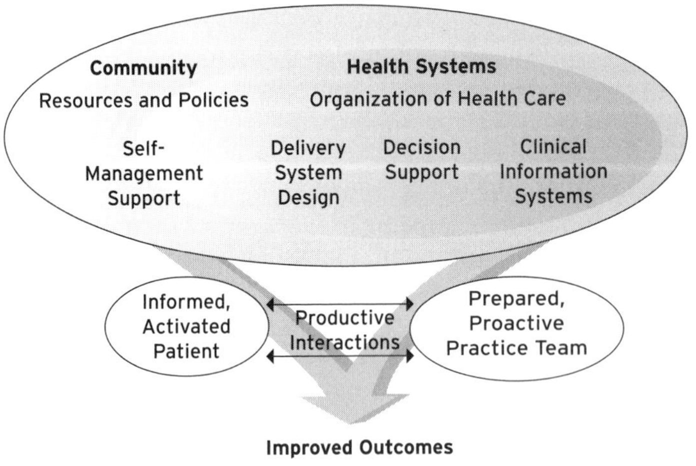

*Source:* Adapted from a figure created by The MacColl Institute ® ACP-ASIM Journals and Books.

foster productive interactions between informed patients who take an active part in their own care and providers with resources and expertise.

Wagner identified a series of key deficiencies in chronic disease management, including clinicians too rushed to spend the time needed with each patient, the failure to apply evidence-based care, the failure to follow up, the failure to coordinate care, and the failure to train patients how best to care for themselves. The Web site for the program Improving Chronic Illness Care (1998) comments that "overcoming these deficiencies will require nothing less than a transformation of health care, from a system that is essentially reactive—responding mainly when a person is sick—to one that is proactive and focused on keeping a person as healthy as possible."

"We were somewhat familiar with Dr. Wagner's model," says Beth Waterman, and she and her physician partner, Dr. John Wheeler, then HealthPartners' associate medical director for primary care, thought it might work for HealthPartners. But they had an even bigger, more powerful idea. What if, they said to their colleagues on the HealthPartners leadership team, we took the Wagner model but rather than applying it only to chronic conditions, we applied it throughout primary care? This was striking and their colleagues immediately liked the idea. They stripped the model down to its essential elements, feeling that might make it more nimble and better applied at the front lines of care. "We needed to make it more straightforward and simple so it would resonate with staff," says Waterman.

## Care Model Process

HealthPartners calls its adaptation of the Wagner chronic care model the Care Model Process. The program goal is to have "prepared practice teams interacting with informed, activated patients through continuous healing relationships supported by the ongoing availability of health information." It is a condition-neutral program focused on shifting from a visit or exam room system to one in which the patient is cared for by a team working collaboratively, caring for patients at all times—before, during, after, and between appointments.

"We redesigned the visit so that we looked at what could happen proactively regardless of condition before the visit took place," says Waterman. She continued:

> So there was previsit planning where the role of the nurse
> was significant. Roles were redefined. Nurses, for example,
> went from . . . rooming patients and thinking of themselves
> as supporting a particular doctor to a much broader role in
> anticipating and serving patient needs. We looked at what could
> happen differently during the visit and changing that interaction.
> And then, particularly with patients with chronic illness, making
> sure that after-visit and between visit care also was part of the
> picture. So with our patients who have chronic conditions,
> [we asked] how could we move to not viewing the exam room as
> the only point of responsibility that we have with those patients and
> what would we do to provide the supportive care before, during,
> and after that interaction?

The Care Model Process was designed to catapult the system past the focus on traditional visit-based care. It required caregivers not only to think of themselves as team members but also to *act* as team members in genuinely collaborative relationships. It also meant educating patients so that nurses, social workers, physician assistants, pharmacists, diabetes educators, and other personnel besides doctors could administer highly valuable care. The actual work of taking the theoretical Wagner model and applying it across primary care was a defining moment in the HealthPartners journey. Figures 1.2 and 1.3 provide a visual definition of the old and new ways at HealthPartners.

## Changing the Way People Work

"If you think about a patient and doctor and a care system coming together, what . . . [does the doctor] know about the patient before they get there?" asks Brian Rank. "What can be done in terms of preventive services, immunizations, labs *before* the visit, etc.?"

At HealthPartners, Rank says, they understand what the science requires in many situations. Guidelines from national organizations

### Figure 1.2. The Old Model of Hierarchy and Autonomy

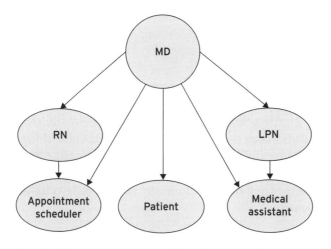

*Source:* Adapted from a figure created by HealthPartners.

### Figure 1.3. The New Model of Patient-Centered Care Using a Prepared Practice Team

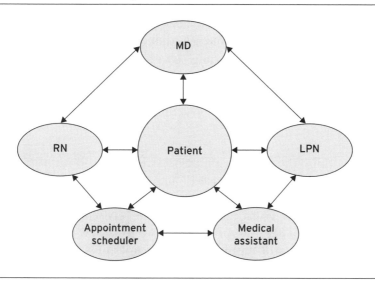

*Source:* Adapted from a figure created by HealthPartners.

and standards from the Institute for Clinical Systems Improvement (a Minnesota collaborative) inform them what works best in many situations. And when a busy primary care doctor is seeing twenty-two to twenty-four patients a day every day, he or she needs reliable systems to support the care team.

In the Care Model Process, every member of the care team works to the limit of his or her license. Thus the physician knows what information gathering and procedures have been covered already by highly reliable members of the team, "and when that physician walks into the exam room . . . [that knowledge] allows the doctor to be a doctor and continue the healing relationship with the patient," says Rank. "Part of the Care Model Process is understanding that human memory is frail and reliable systems are far better."

The process also requires "engineering the after visit," says Rank:

> [P]atients in the highly emotionally charged experience [of the visit] don't remember much of what we say so the after-visit summary is in writing and the patient takes it with them. Then there is engineering the between visit care, for example, reaching out to patients to make sure they are on their medications. The Care Model Process is about reliably coordinating all of those things. It means engineering reliability and safety into our clinics and hospitals. It means coming up with ideas on how to establish the best transfer from the hospital to outpatient care. It is an incredibly complex world in health care and we can do a lot better by working together and constructing those supports at the point of care.

Essentially, the Care Model Process is "really about how we do our work," says Dr. Rae Ann Williams, a HealthPartners medical director for primary care. "At the time of the visit certain things need to be done consistently when the physician is seeing the patient, and it is also the physician's job to review preventive services. The nurse will highlight, for example, if a patient doesn't want to do a colonoscopy or doesn't want to do a mammogram, and that is a chance for the physician and the patient to have that conversation about the preventive services recommendations."

The Care Model Process is about reliability, patient centered-ness, and standardization. The approach leverages electronic medical records to help make sure that all recommended care is identified and delivered at every visit. Rank and the leader-ship team identified the following design principles on which the Care Model Process is built:

- Use existing staff.
- Use no added resources.
- Start small.
- Make it condition neutral.
- Ensure that the right person is doing the right work.
- Increase provider efficiency.
- Support the patient-provider relationship.
- Establish joint accountability.

Nancy McClure notes that HealthPartners is constantly making efforts "to incorporate improvement in our process. We do this by working with our care teams and the patient to upgrade the Care Model Process, a familiar concept from the technology world."

## Building Reliability and Redundancy into the Clinic Setting

The Care Model Process builds "reliability with a redundancy component into the clinic setting," says Dr. Beth Averbeck, asso-ciate medical director for primary care, by assigning specific roles and responsibilities for all members of the clinical team. Primary care, she says, is "a team sport and you have to trust your team—nurses, pharmacists, diabetes educators, everybody."

The workflow begins a week before a patient visit, when a nurse reviews the schedule and orders whatever preparation is needed—labs, screenings, and so forth. A member of the clinical team calls the patient and offers him or her the opportunity to come in prior to the appointment so the labs can be completed in time for that session (though this is not mandatory). There is a redundant step when the patient arrives and the schedule is reviewed again for any orders needed. The team also identifies patients who have not filled prescriptions or will soon need to fill them.

The "Care Model Process is standardizing how to do care," says Dr. David Caccamo, a primary care physician in the HealthPartners Cottage Grove clinic, "patients can expect reliable, standard, high-quality care wherever they go in the system." And as the new approach has become deeply ingrained in HealthPartners in recent years, Caccamo says, there is a very different attitude among clinicians: "People have a systems mentality now that they didn't have before."

## Improving Access

No matter how solid the new approach was in theory, however, it would not have worked without easy access to appointments. "Access was a big challenge for us," says Brainerd.

> We had lousy access in both primary care and specialty so that was really a foundational change that we needed to make. We had a lot of infrastructure work getting our patients in the door. In confronting access we confronted a lot of the really daunting issues around standardization—standardization of appointment types— actually creating access. We need to do what it takes to make sure the patients can get in to see us. Over time, the concept has broadened to include more convenient and affordable methods including e-visits and phone visits. We call this "call, click, or come in."

A service created by HealthPartners called *virtuwell* enables patients to get online treatment for more than forty common conditions, ranging from the flu to a sinus infection.

## Increasing Coordination

In addition to access, coordination was foundational to the new Care Model Process, and Brainerd has a unique view of coordination because she has seen it both as CEO and as a patient. "I have a personal story that is a big driver for me," she says.

> A number of years ago I was diagnosed with breast cancer and I went to the oncologist, surgeon, and the radiation oncologist, all of whom had slightly different recommendations for follow up. Well,

as a patient what that leaves you with is, "I don't know who to trust, I don't know who to believe and why aren't these people talking to each other?"

I think we have come a long way in having a consumer perspective even in terms of basic clinical information. We have just created a common, reliable pathway across all the related specialties (thoracic surgery, pulmonary, oncology) and primary care for our patients who have a lung nodule or cancer so they get the same message every time from every provider because . . . [these specialists] created the pathway together. In a fragmented system this coordination doesn't happen and the message to the patient varies from provider to provider. Think about what that does to a patient. We can do so much better.

## Standardizing *Then* Customizing

HealthPartners has learned that standardization is really part of a two-step process. "When you work on standardization," says McClure, "there is always this backlash, 'Well, that's cookie-cutter medicine,' and it's played out as an either-or. *Either we are going to personalize care or we are going to standardize.* But we see standardization and customization working together. First, design reliable systems and processes, and *then and only then* we customize to individual patient preferences, values, or changes in clinical guidelines." An example of how this can work has to do with the recommended age for screening African American and Native American patients for colorectal cancer.

Since 2004, HealthPartners has gathered data from patients on race and language, for the purpose of identifying disparities in care and filling those gaps. Very few provider organizations collect such data, but for many years HealthPartners has viewed this information as an essential element for dealing with racial disparities in care, and for certain patients it has proved immensely valuable, perhaps even life saving. For instance, the guidelines indicate that for African American and Native American patients with average risk factors, screening for colorectal cancer should start at age forty-five, not age fifty as is the case for the rest of the population. Because HealthPartners can identify the ethnicity of its patients, the alert in the electronic medical records of its African American and Native American patients now calls for this screening at age forty-five.

McClure cites this as an example of customization on a standardized platform. "Another example," she says, "is breast cancer screening. We found when we collected data on our screening rates by race that women of color were not screened at the same rate as women who are white. Our system prompts us to send reminders to patients and that works for a lot of women. But we found that for some women, particularly newer Americans who are less familiar with preventive care, this doesn't work as well. So, we designed a redundancy step." And here is where standardization allows flexibility. When a patient overdue for a mammogram comes to the clinic for another reason, the patient is offered an opportunity to have a mammogram right then and there— guaranteed within an hour and usually much faster. The radiology teams, knowing how crucial and life saving it can be, are energized by the work. HealthPartners has been doing an average of 500 same-day mammographies per month, with 150 of these in the high-risk group of women aged fifty to seventy-five and overdue for screening. This effort has narrowed the gap between white women and women of color for mammogram screenings from 12.4 percent in 2007 to 4.9 percent in late 2011, and the screening rate for women of color at HealthPartners exceeds the rate for all women achieved by organizations in the HEDIS (Healthcare Effectiveness Data and Information Set) ninetieth percentile.

How big a deal are standardization, reliability, and customization at HealthPartners?

McClure: "Oh, it is everything."

Rank: "It is our foundation."

## Piloting Flow Stations

The Care Model Process has worked well. In 2004 at HealthPartners, a total of 8 percent of all visits were preplanned. By 2009, it was 96 percent. One glitch, however, was that clinical teams found themselves perpetually running behind. When they stepped back and measured, they found that their twenty-minute clinic appointments actually ran twenty-three minutes.

To help solve that problem, HealthPartners' clinical teams are piloting the primary care flow stations developed by the primary care teams at Virginia Mason. Dr Laurel Morrison of VM Kirkland was the first to trial this method of unbatching lab results, prescriptions, phone care and medical forms. During a week-long process improvement workshop, this Virginia Mason team set up simple flow stations outside the exam rooms, where a physician and medical assistant work side by side throughout the day. Each flow station has two computers, a phone, and designated areas for paperwork generated throughout the course of a day. Pittenger and his colleagues found that on average, in the course of a typical primary care doctor's day, three pieces of paper were generated per visit. So a physician seeing twenty patients would have about sixty pieces of paper awaiting his or her attention at day's end. This was the major reason why doctors at Virginia Mason were staying late, were taking work home, and were less than satisfied with their work-life balance.

Working within the flow station, all that has changed. The medical assistant manages the flow of paper in real time and is empowered to make many decisions that do not require a doctor's expertise. The physician, instead of batching the work for the end of the day, deals with it in real time between visits throughout the day. This approach, which has now spread throughout the Virginia Mason primary care clinics, has succeeded in helping physicians get nearly all of their paperwork done during the course of normal business hours so that they can walk out the door on time and head home.

This real-time attention to the work also provides better, more patient-centered care. It means tests are ordered more quickly, results are processed faster, and patients get whatever they need—information, medicines, and so forth—more rapidly. And the flow station process has significantly reduced the possibility of human error that existed with batching.

In the HealthPartners clinics where flow stations are being piloted, they have thus far worked well. If this result holds up, Beth Averbeck will be spreading them throughout the HealthPartners primary care system. "Using flow stations just ramps up the Care Model Process," she says, and it will allow primary care doctors to shave that three minutes off so that a twenty-minute appointment can be achieved in twenty minutes rather than twenty-three.

## Addressing Cultural Change

The changes required to make the Care Model Process work were significant. Many were structural of course, but among the most critical was cultural change and cultural change meant making a compelling case to physicians that they should not only support the new approach but embrace it. "Both physicians and the leadership team together were saying we need to address this thing called culture," says Rank. And that would involve an examination of what HealthPartners' existing culture really was and what sort of cultural shifts might be needed to create a new form of care.

Dr. George Isham, chief health officer for HealthPartners, says the organization has

> a value system that relates to thinking consistently in terms of teamwork, that it is not OK for the different specialties among the doctors to fight with each other. It is not okay for the health plan to beat up on the medical group or vice versa. We are a team and we need to make that work. We have to have trust and respect for each other to make that happen. Those are all the kinds of values that I think are important for us to hold in common and reinforce and so we work pretty hard at doing that.

Perhaps that is why Rank believed the process of working out a physician compact would be relatively straightforward. "In my naiveté, I thought this was going to be a really easy discussion," says Rank. But, as hospitals and physician practices throughout the country have consistently found, it is anything but easy.

Conversations among doctors and between doctors and the HealthPartners leadership were initiated and sustained over many months. "We recognized that as doctors, each of us had been creating our own processes, which for our own practice was somewhat reliable, yet when we measured we found wide variation in outcomes," says Rank. "Doctors did what we needed to do to get through the day, but we had to understand there is variation in outcomes with that approach. The Care Model Process was about creating reliable supporting processes across our care."

Doctors had been creating their own processes for varying lengths of time—some had finished their residencies or fellowships in the seventies, others in the eighties, the nineties, or more recently. But generally none of them had been taught during their years of education and training, that standardization was an essential component for reliability. Atul Gawande made this point in his Harvard commencement address in which he talked about certain skills the graduates would need but would have not been taught, such as

> the ability to implement at scale, the ability to get colleagues along the entire chain of care functioning like pit crews for patients. There is resistance, sometimes vehement resistance, to the efforts that make it possible. Partly, it is because the work is rooted in different values than the ones we've had. They include humility, an understanding that no matter who you are, how experienced or smart, you will fail. They include discipline, the belief that standardization, doing certain things the same way every time, can reduce your failures. And they include teamwork, the recognition that others can save you from failure, no matter who they are in the hierarchy.

The cultural shift required an acceptance by doctors that standardization and reliability were essential elements of delivering quality care.

Rank notes that in American health care delivery "the concept of reliability science is almost brand new. And the science of care improvement is pretty young as well. Having these concepts in front of doctors—that you are part of a team and you can be supported and the system in which you work can make you a better or worse doctor—our training programs in medical schools don't understand that. As a result doctors throughout the United States believed they must reinvent their own wheels time after time after time."

In all, the cultural dialogue took a year and a half and was finally completed in November 2006. The result was the HealthPartners Physician & Dentist Partnership Agreement, a one-page document that described an ideal relationship through a list of organizational *gives* and physician and dentist *gives*. Among the more than two dozen items included under physician *gives* were the following: "pursue clinical practice consistent with the 6 Aims," "seek and implement best practices of care for patients," and "reduce unnecessary variation in care to support quality reliability, and customized care based on patients' needs." In a way this was the heart of the agreement, for it got at the idea of standardization as promoted in *Crossing the Quality Chasm*—and away from the kind of autonomy that made for unnecessary variation in the delivery and outcomes of care.

"It was all about how we create the kind of care embodied in the *Quality Chasm*," says Rank. "You don't build a reliable and standardized system of care without working through cultural change. The partnership agreement set a tone that we are all in this together and that we approach each other by assuming good intent and that we all want what is best for the patient."

When the partnership agreement was completed, Rank and everyone else wanted to be sure it didn't sit on a shelf gathering dust. "One of the things we heard from our doctors was, 'sometimes you hire people who don't fit our culture and it really sends an inconsistent message,' so we all wanted the partnership to be a key part of the hiring process," says Rank.

Rank personally interviews every physician who is a serious candidate for a position, and he goes through a process. "I talk with every physician coming in and tell them who we are and what we strive for to let them know what we expect and what they can expect from us," he says. "Physicians I interview are often very happy to hear that someone is paying attention to this." He gives each doctor three documents: the partnership agreement, the *Chasm* executive summary, and the Reinertsen article about physician autonomy.

Rank has been using this approach for some years because he and his colleagues believe so strongly that these elements are essential pieces of HealthPartners' intellectual and practical foundation. "Unfortunately, most residencies and practices haven't incorporated the design principles in *Crossing the Quality Chasm* into their training programs and care," he says. "I think I interview between two hundred and three hundred doctors per year, and I would say less than 1 percent have even heard of this transformational document."

## Diabetes: An Optimal Measure

As early as 1999, Dr. Gail Amundson, former medical director for quality and improvement at HealthPartners, sought to develop an "all or nothing" composite measure for diabetes and coronary artery disease. Mary Brainerd says it is important to pursue aggressive goals in chronic conditions, given how crucial it is to a patient's well-being to keep his or her conditions under control. Thus the creation at HealthPartners of the *optimal diabetes measure.*

Under this measure, care teams and patients with diabetes work toward meeting five targets to prevent medical complications such as amputations, heart attacks, and blindness. The optimal diabetes measure is recognized as not only one of the most challenging measures in the country, but also one of the most effective—so much so that the Institute of Medicine has suggested that all providers adopt it for patients with diabetes. The five targets, or goals, are

- Hemoglobin A1c $\leq$ 7.9
- Low-density lipoprotein $\leq$ 99
- Blood pressure $\leq$ 139/89
- Non-tobacco user
- Regular aspirin user

The measure sets a high bar. If a patient meets the goals on four of the five items in the measure, he or she does not meet the standard—only those patients who achieve all five meet it.

Brainerd wanted transparency. She felt she owed it to patients, and she knew it would intensify competition among clinicians and thus drive results. She wanted the entire organization to set an aggressive goal and reveal the results—whatever those results happened to be. Transparency in health care can sometimes be quite painful and that was surely the case with the initial results from the optimal diabetes measure. "We don't have poor results very often any more but that was not true when we first started" with the diabetes measure, says Brainerd. "There were some times it was really sad to see where we were. I remember when we started measuring our optimal diabetes results and thought we were hitting on all cylinders and only 5 percent of our patients met the optimal measure. That was a sorry day."

But through the concerted work of primary care teams using the Care Model Process and engaging patients, the results improved steadily over time to the point where, in the summer of 2011, more than 42 percent of HealthPartners' patients with diabetes met all five measures. And the trend continues upward (Figure 1.4). Some providers at HealthPartners clinics—working relentlessly with excellent teams—have reached the point where 65 percent of their patients with diabetes meet all five measures. David Caccamo and his team, for example, have over 66 percent of their patients routinely hitting all five marks.

"Our teams engage patients so that if you have diabetes and you are missing something we create supports for you to get to the next level," says Brian Rank. "We know our patients live longer and have a better quality of life if they achieve control over blood sugar, blood pressure, lipids, don't smoke, and take an aspirin each day. We have 13,800 patients with diabetes and

## Figure 1.4. Optimal Diabetes Measure, 2004 to 2011

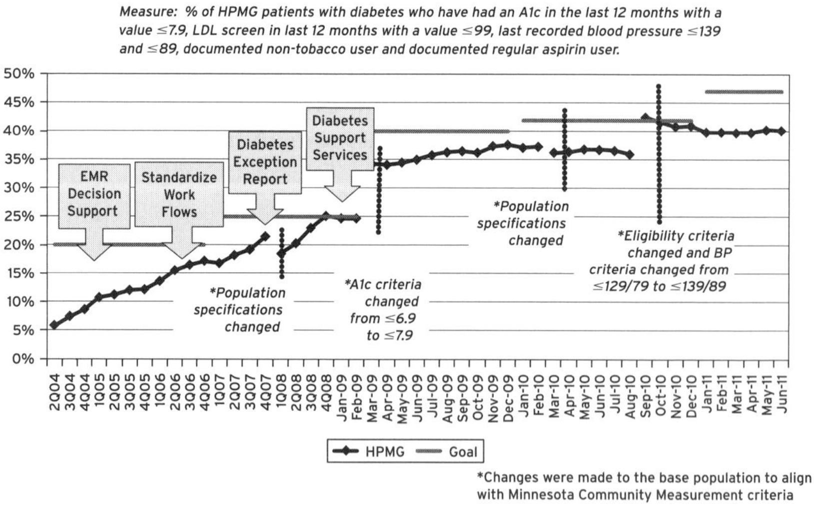

Measure: % of HPMG patients with diabetes who have had an A1c in the last 12 months with a value ≤7.9, LDL screen in last 12 months with a value ≤99, last recorded blood pressure ≤139 and ≤89, documented non-tobacco user and documented regular aspirin user.

*Changes were made to the base population to align with Minnesota Community Measurement criteria

*Source:* Figure created by HealthPartners.

we routinely know where each patient is in terms of their optimal care measure, and its transparency becomes a tool for the patient and the care team."

This diabetes work affects both quality and cost. When the teams manage patients with diabetes effectively, the costs of care average about $1,500 per year. For patients with poorly managed diabetes, the annual cost is $20,000. Indeed, compared to HealthPartners members who fail to get all the recommended care for their diabetes, those who do get all this care suffered 364 fewer heart attacks ($35,000 per episode), 68 fewer leg amputations ($26,000 per episode), and 625 fewer eye complications, which may lead to blindness ($250 to $3,000 per episode). In addition, there were 1,200 fewer emergency department (ED) visits in one year among patients with diabetes who participated in the HealthPartners diabetes disease management program compared to those who did not participate. The average ED visit costs $750, so avoiding 1,200 visits reduced costs by $900,000 (HealthPartners, 2011).

To achieve results such as these requires reliable, timely, actionable data. Every month HealthPartners primary care teams receive up-to-date data on where each patient stands on the five goals. Overall results for each group are also posted online. This not only enables patients to compare groups but also fosters a healthy sense of competition among the groups.

## Teamwork, Teamwork, Teamwork

"Five or six years ago we dealt with chronic care with the brute force of the doctor in the exam room," Caccamo says. "You could only get so far and it was not far enough." Thus Caccamo set out to improve what he calls the "*teamness* of how we did our diabetes work." Working in collaboration with a nurse, medical assistant, diabetes educator (usually a nurse), and pharmacist, the Caccamo team pored through the data, identifying patients who did not have the basics covered. A nurse then called these patients and urged them to come in for their labs.

Caccamo and his colleagues have established several categories for their patients: at goal, near goal, more distant from goal, and unengaged. Those at goal receive reminder calls at appropriate times from the clinic receptionist. For patients near goal, an RN makes a detailed assessment of what the patient needs. Patients more distant from goal are addressed by the care team at a monthly care management conference where team members review the patient list and make a plan for each individual. Team members then follow up with their different functions throughout the week. Nurses call with reminders about tests and medications. Diabetes educators meet one-on-one with patients in the office or discuss issues by phone. Pharmacists work with patients on blood pressure guidelines and medication adjustments. Every call is scripted: *I am working with your doctor; we do this as a team . . .*

With unengaged patients, Caccamo's team makes sure they are offered opportunities to get engaged, including suggestions for making office visits, for getting lab work done, and so on. But with this patient population no progress was possible until the patient decided to act.

The HealthPartners teams found there is both art and science to the diabetes work. The science centers on the measurement of the types of medicines and best practices for controlling blood pressure, blood sugars, and so on. But there is also a great deal of art to the work in such areas as engaging effectively with patients and determining the right medications at the right dosage.

Blood pressure, the most important of the risk factors, presents particular challenges. When a patient is diagnosed with diabetes, says Caccamo, "it often means more medicines, sometimes increasing doses and adding new single drugs or combination medicines. Usually two to three medications are required to control blood pressure in patients with diabetes—the average is something like 2.7." Caccamo finds that clinical pharmacists do an excellent job of working with patients to identify medications that minimize side effects and the number of pills that must be taken each day. This is critical because "the number of pills is a barrier for patients," says Caccamo, "and cost is a barrier as well." Thus when the team works effectively with a patient to minimize the number of pills and the cost, adherence by patients increases.

Reaching the LDL (low-density lipoprotein) target level typically requires the use of statins. Again, this is an area where the pharmacist plays an important team role by integrating blood pressure and cholesterol medicines. Many patients are brought to this goal by effective use of medications and diet, and it is not unusual to have a patient with diabetes whose LDL level is quite high—north of 200, for example—who responds well to statins. "Even if their cholesterol levels can't be brought down all the way to the goal, we know that the treatment we do offer still has a big impact on their risk of heart disease," Caccamo says. "Some patients come from an LDL of 210 to 120 or so, and even though they are not under 100 and have not reached goal, they are much better off, much healthier."

Controlling blood sugar is again part art and part science, with both medications and vigilant management playing important roles. Clinicians have choices of numerous different oral medications as well as injectable insulin.

## Every Team Member a Respected Expert

Caccamo puts patients newly diagnosed with diabetes on a program and quickly brings in other team members. New patients benefit significantly from time with a diabetes educator. Says Caccamo, "I am an expert in this but the other team members are experts too. The diabetes educator is very good at using insulin and in recognizing blood sugar patterns and helping patients make medication adjustments to improve their sugars. When I have patients struggling with sugars I send them to the diabetes educator."

The only one of the five targets in the optimal measure that cannot be measured particularly well is aspirin use. It is a self-reported metric, so the team must take the word of patients when they say they are in fact taking their aspirin regularly.

The toughest of the five targets to deal with, of course, is tobacco use. Caccamo says that for patients with diabetes, not smoking is just about as important as controlling blood pressure but vastly more difficult to achieve. "Smoking is a different beast," he says. But he finds that if the team is able to make some progress with a patient in other areas, say blood pressure or cholesterol, that patient will then sometimes turn his or her attention and energy to quitting smoking.

"The key is we don't give up," says Rae Ann Williams. "We realize that it is really tough to change. I met with a physician leader who has a smoking rate of 40 percent in her patients with diabetes. I said to her, 'let's not look at that. You will deal with that when they come in but let's look at the other components. We know smoking is going to affect your optimal diabetes outcome, but let's look at the opportunities in LDL and A1c and blood pressure because there are still opportunities there.'"

Clearly, when a patient with diabetes smokes, the optimal measure remains unmet, even if that patient is perfect on the other four goals. But that doesn't mean you should despair, says Williams. There are various ways to look at progress apart from fixing on the optimal measure's bottom-line number. And Williams points out that even as clinicians work diligently toward smoking cessation, they also say it is useful to look at other components presenting an opportunity for improvement.

Although the HealthPartners average on achieving the optimal diabetes measure stands at 42 percent, some provider teams have reached the mid-60s, which Caccamo believes is about as high as it is possible to achieve. "The maximum you can get depends on the teamwork, how skilled the team is, and how skilled the doctor is also," he says. Indeed, although physician leadership is crucial, there are indications that some teams are extremely skilled at this work. Caccamo says that when one particular doctor took a six-month sabbatical, she met with her team before leaving and encouraged them to continue good work on diabetes. Overall, her patients had a very high score on the optimal measure and she was hoping the team would be able to sustain it until she returned. The team did better than that: when she returned she found they had improved the score!

Outcomes on the optimal measure also depend of course on the population being managed. An affluent, well-educated population of patients with diabetes is likely to reach higher scores than a population that is in a different demographic range.

Williams agrees with Caccamo that there is no single strategy or approach that works in diabetes care, unless it is relying on a coordinated effort by all clinical team members. "Physicians alone cannot do this work," she says. "It is about using your care team, clinical pharmacist, your diabetic nurse educator, using your nurse to help with that outreach, so there is not one strategy that works. Before we had a team-based approach, it would have really been left to the physician, and if the patient came into the office for a visit, we would address their diabetes. But a patient could have easily not come in and we then would not be making a move on their medication to try to get them within goal."

## Diabetes Wizard and the EHR

Rae Ann Williams says a critical aspect of diabetes improvement work is sustaining the effort with patients who, for a wide variety of reasons, are not reaching goal. Sometimes the difficulty is inertia on the part of the patient, but Williams says it is often inertia on the part of the care team. Several years ago the HealthPartners Research Foundation conducted a study (funded by the National Institute of Diabetes and Digestive and Kidney Diseases) that found that a relatively simple tool—dubbed the Diabetes Wizard—could improve performance among patients with diabetes.

Diabetes Wizard is now built into the electronic medical record and helps to guide clinicians in their decision making about what treatments might be best for patients. It allows clinicians to both standardize and personalize care using a single tool and has resulted in significantly better glucose and blood pressure control in those patients whose providers are using it. Mary Brainerd says the beauty of Diabetes Wizard is that it identifies the right treatments for patients with diabetes, customized to the specific interventions best suited to their needs.

HealthPartners' use of Diabetes Wizard was included in a study conducted by Sperl-Hillen et al. and discussed in *Diabetes Spectrum* in 2010. This study found "that 'clinical inertia,' defined as failure to intensify drug therapy at a clinical encounter when the patient is not at the recommended clinical goals, is a second major barrier to better diabetes care," in addition to patient noncompliance. Indeed, this and "other head-to-head studies suggest that clinical inertia is a bigger problem than patient nonadherence." In investigating ways of overcoming clinical inertia in the primary care setting, Sperl-Hillen et al. (2010) found that electronic health records (EHRs) could play a key role in managing patients with diabetes, particularly when combined with a clinical decision support tool such as Diabetes Wizard.

These authors noted that this tool was adopted in six randomly selected HealthPartners clinics in 2007 and that primary care teams "reported high levels of satisfaction with the tool, in terms of both its clinical content and its user interface . . . [and that] preliminary results appear quite favorable." In discussing the Diabetes Wizard and its incorporation into the EHR, some members of the HealthPartners leadership team made the point that even though electronic health records are essential for employing tools like the wizard, there is broad recognition within HealthPartners that EHRs by themselves do not solve anything; that they must be used in strategic and purposeful ways within the broader care process. HealthPartners experimented with EHRs back in the 1990s (the first beta site was 1996). In a pilot project the primary care clinic using electronic records performed no better than any other HealthPartners clinic.

"It was a perfect case in point where just having the EMR does not necessarily lead to better outcomes," says Beth Waterman. "When we implemented it fully we probably did it in the wrong order because we did it right before the Care Model Process rollout. Ideally we would have built the workflows first. You want the workflows to drive the electronic medical record, not the other way around."

## Evolving to the Triple Aim

When David Caccamo, working in his clinic some miles from the HealthPartners headquarters, is asked what the Triple Aim has to do with his practice, he laughs as though the answer could not be more obvious. "It has *everything* do with it," he replies.

When IHI launched the Triple Aim initiative in 2007, the goal was to help organizations simultaneously improve the experience of care by providing safe, effective, reliable care to every patient, every time; improve the health of a population by focusing on prevention and wellness; and decrease per capita costs. HealthPartners leaders saw this as a logical evolution of the six aims they had adopted from *Crossing the Quality Chasm*, recognizing that all six are essentially embedded in the Triple Aim.

"The Triple Aim crystallized the issue of value," says Mary Brainerd. "We must improve the health of the population and the experience of care, but we need to do it in a way that makes things more affordable. We felt like cost showed up in the six aims in efficiency and effectiveness but it was still a little bit hidden." So at about that time, HealthPartners shifted its language and began talking about using the Triple Aim rather the six aims.

Since that time, HealthPartners has spread the Care Model Process design principles of reliability, customization, access, and coordination across all areas of its delivery system. An example of how this plays out in practice is the current care for back pain. HealthPartners has implemented an evidence-based best practice for conservative treatment of back pain across primary and specialty care. "We have concentrated our efforts on areas where we see a real return on the Triple Aim," says Nancy McClure.

Brian Rank adds that "the idea is to do all of these things not just in silos of primary care and the hospital, but seamlessly across the continuum of care."

## Functioning as a Medical Home and an ACO

With primary care redesign and the Triple Aim at the heart of clinicians' work, HealthPartners is particularly well positioned as both a *medical home* and an *accountable care organization* (ACO). These approaches do not require any significant change in the organization's care delivery model. In fact they are so consistent with what HealthPartners is doing that they can be properly viewed as evolutions of the HealthPartners process. (HealthPartners was the first health care system in the United States to have all of its clinics secure the medical home designation at the highest level from the National Committee for Quality Assurance.)

"We are ready to participate in ACO payment models," says Nancy McClure, "but we are spending the bulk of our time on redesigning our systems so that we can reliably produce Triple Aim results. If the system can't deliver results, it won't matter what kind of ACO contract we enter into." George Isham (2011) has written that with its integrated health plan, hospitals, and medical group, HealthPartners "already operates in many ways as a self-contained ACO." In the same article, he noted that accountable care organizations are designed to address "the fragmented, disconnected nature of fee for service health care delivery in most parts of the United States—and the ways in which it rewards volume instead of results. . . . In practice, an ACO should allow hospitals, clinics, administrators and clinicians to work together—usually across systems—to address challenges in planned, measurable ways." Just as HealthPartners does.

## A Health *Behavior* Problem More Than a Health *Care* Problem

Prevention and wellness—the population piece of the Triple Aim—is at the core of what HealthPartners is aiming for in the years ahead. Brainerd and Rank note that "four lifestyle behaviors could avoid 25 percent of health care costs: healthy diet (five servings of fruits/vegetables/day); regular exercise; not smoking; avoiding risky alcohol use." They also note a particularly sobering statistic: that as of 2009, a total of 8.6 percent of HealthPartners members met all four of these lifestyle goals.

HealthPartners cardiologist Dr. Thomas Kottke and Nico Pronk, two behavioral and population health specialists at HealthPartners, are intensively focused on the population health leg of the Triple Aim, an area they have been working in for many years. An important aspect of that work has focused on employers. "Working with employers has been the best way to get the reach and frequency of messages to members that is needed," Kottke says. "In a couple of key groups, more than 90 percent of employees are taking health assessments, and nearly 60 percent have been involved in prevention programs." Pronk points out that they "have been able to document that employer-based wellness programs, supported by strong communications and incentives, can make an impressive impact on healthiness, reduce cost, and increase productivity."

Pronk believes it is much more challenging to do prevention and wellness work in a primary care clinic setting than in the workplace where there is a clearly defined population "and you have extended exposure to people and we can stay with them for long periods of time. It gives us an opportunity to interact much more intensively over time with the same people."

Most of the HealthPartners workplace programs target behavioral change such as tobacco use, exercise, and weight management. There is also help and support for management of chronic conditions. Typically, when HealthPartners goes into a company it helps the employer create incentives for employees to participate and communicates aggressively with employees about the program and its potential benefits.

"We identify the level of risk people have and we look at specific risk for diabetes and heart disease," says Pronk. "Many of the risk factors are behavioral and therefore modifiable." The programs that do best, says Pronk, are those where there is an incentive built into the process, "so that if you do a health assessment and participate in follow-up you get a break on your deductible and co-pay." The work is done one employer at a time, thus enabling the HealthPartners team to dig in and understand the needs of that employer.

HealthPartners is now exploring how to better integrate this work into the clinic visit. "We've been piloting a health assessment that the patient can have sent to the doctor before the visit," says Beth Averbeck. "This gives us a chance to engage the patient in a conversation about behavior change, and we are training our care teams in basic health coaching skills."

## Collaboration and Transparency

HealthPartners has a long history of collaboration. Since the early 1990s, HealthPartners has worked in concert with the Mayo Clinic, Park Nicollet Health Services, and others to create a unique collaborative focused on identifying best practices and measuring results. The Institute for Clinical Systems Improvement (ICSI) has become a nationally recognized center of expertise on evidence-based guidelines, improvement practices, and measurement. The result is that "Minnesota became the first state in the nation where medical care was built around the systematic use of science-based best medical practices developed by physicians and sponsored by major health plans" (Institute for Clinical Systems Improvement, 2010).

"How do you create a standard?" asks Brian Rank, who in addition to his leadership role at HealthPartners also serves as chair of the ICSI board of directors. "What does the evidence show, and how do we put that into an algorithm and processes that can support teams, doctors, and patients in improving care? How do we synthesize the world literature for clinicians?'" Answering those sorts of questions is what ICSI is all about. The organization includes more than sixty medical groups that represent an estimated 85 percent of the doctors in Minnesota. And Nancy McClure notes that the major health plans have embraced ICSI standards "so we don't have different health plans with different standards or different measurement systems by and large." Brian Rank says the ICSI is all about providing evidence-based guidelines that help a clinician deliver the best possible care. And ICSI has now declared that the Triple Aim has become its "guidepost."

Along with its history of collaboration, HealthPartners has a tradition of measuring and transparently reporting results, and it is one of the founders of Minnesota Community Measurement, the state's measurement collaborative that is supported by all care systems and plans in Minnesota. The results of the Care Model Process can be seen in the 2010 Minnesota Community Measurement report in which HealthPartners Medical Group had results with confidence intervals above the state average for ten of the eleven measures (Figure 1.5)—the best results among all the large care delivery systems in the state.

## The Future

HealthPartners continues to set ambitious goals as it looks to the future for transformation. The leaders are currently working on the Partners for Better Health Goals 2014, which are focused on the three objectives of the Triple Aim and which include the following:

Health success: improved health for customers and community as measured by

- Better well-being, more satisfied and healthy lives
- The best local and national health outcomes and the best performing health costs in the region

## Figure 1.5. Minnesota Community Measures: High-Performing Medical Groups in 2010, Primary Care

| Medical Group | Asthma | Upper Respiratory Infection | Pharyngitis | Bronchitis | Optimal Diabetes | Optimal Vascular | Controlling High BP | Colorectal Cancer Screening | Breast Cancer Screening | Cervical Cancer Screening | Cancer Screening Combined | Chlamydia Screening | Childhood Immunization Status | COPD |
|---|---|---|---|---|---|---|---|---|---|---|---|---|---|---|
| HealthPartners Clinics 12 out of 14 | | ● | ● | | ● | ● | ● | ● | ● | ● | ● | ● | ● | ● |
| Park Nicollet Health Services 9 out of 14 | | ● | ● | | ● | ● | ● | | ● | ● | | | ● | ● |
| Quello Clinic 9 out of 14 | | | | | ● | ● | ● | ● | ● | ● | ● | ● | ⊘ | ● |
| CentraCare Health System 8 out of 14 | ● | ● | | | ● | ● | | ● | ● | ● | ● | | | |
| HealthEast 8 out of 14 | | ● | ● | | ● | ● | ● | ● | | | | ● | ● | |
| Fairview Health Services 8 out of 14 | | ● | ● | ● | ● | ● | | | | ● | ● | ● | | |

●- Medical group rate and fully above state average
⊘- Data size too small
Blank - Measure reported but rate was average or below average.

*Source:* Figure created by HealthPartners.

Experience: delivery of an exceptional experience that customers want and deserve at an affordable cost as measured by

- The best performance on customer's willingness to recommend HealthPartners clinics, hospitals, and health plan to family and friends
- Feeling well supported, respected, and cared for throughout life

Affordability: lower health care costs for customers as measured by

- Cost trends that are at or below the CPI
- The best-performing overall health care costs in the region
- HealthPartners clinics and hospitals being in the best 10 percent in the region in overall costs of health care

George Isham has been at HealthPartners for twenty-one years and he has an excellent perspective on where the organization has been and where it is headed. "Over time, we have been able to improve care for people with diabetes very significantly," he says. "We have been able to reduce our relative cost of care in this market by a significant amount. We have contributed to the reduction in mortality rates for cardiovascular disease in Minnesota—now our cardiovascular mortality rates are lower relative to cardiovascular rates of mortality in most other states. Being organized as we are at HealthPartners enables us to achieve these broader and very significant outcomes in the health of Minnesotans in addition to being able to provide outstanding individual clinical care."

## Keys to Doing This Work

HealthPartners' leaders generously share their ideas for improvement. They believe that an organization wishing to adopt some of their best practices requires the following key elements for a successful redesign of its care process.

- **A clear vision.** A clear, shared vision among the board members and senior leaders is essential. Progress toward the vision requires setting ambitious goals and transparently reporting results.
- **A Triple Aim focus.** Measuring progress on all three elements of the Triple Aim simultaneously is a powerful way to keep an organization on track.
- **The right leadership structure.** The HealthPartners leadership system pairs an administrative leader and a physician leader in each area. The two manage their areas as a team, agreeing on all decisions before any changes are made. This unites the two sometimes quite different administrative and clinical points

of view. Together, "they see the whole picture," says Beth Waterman.

- **Design principles.** In order to practice design with intention, HealthPartners applies its set of design principles across the system: reliability, customization, access, and coordination. The EHR is essential, but it is not sufficient on its own to drive change.
- **Cultural change.** The cultural change required to succeed with team-based medicine is considerable. For HealthPartners this change was a long and not altogether easy process but nonetheless essential. The organizational culture needs not only to accept standardization and reliability but also to embrace them, to act every day on the belief that the center of the HealthPartners universe is the patient and not the provider.
- **Involvement of patients and families.** As Nancy McClure says, "We've found it really changes the focus of the discussion to have a patient involved."
- **Teamwork.** The Care Process Model works, in part, because the teams are working in new ways to have individuals working to their full capabilities, to huddle and design care together, and in new roles and new communication processes.

# 2

# Intel and Virginia Mason Medical Center

## Marketplace Collaboratives for Better, Faster, More Affordable Care

What if American companies used their marketplace clout to demand a certain level of quality from health care providers? What if these companies—individually and collectively—insisted on adherence to performance standards for high-quality care for the medical conditions that have the greatest impact on their employees' health and their company's bottom line? What if companies managed health care services the way they manage all other suppliers, with intense rigor and clear parameters? This chapter focuses on these ideas as they were applied by Virginia Mason Medical Center and by Intel—with surprising and encouraging results. The work outlined here indicates a pathway to significant gains in the health of workers in a variety of employment settings—improvements that are pivotal to achieving the Triple Aim. What's more, the work also demonstrates quite clearly that better care can also come at a lower cost when waste is eliminated.

The foundation for this work was built when Dr. Gary Kaplan, CEO of Virginia Mason Medical Center in Seattle, led his team in adapting Toyota Production System methods to health care, creating what they call the Virginia Mason Production System. The Toyota system was steeped in the idea of *lean* manufacturing, and lean tools and methods were to become central to Virginia Mason's new system. Beginning in 2001, Kaplan led an effort to identify waste in the Virginia Mason system, to provide full transparency around that waste, and to eliminate it. This was a remarkable effort that empowered clinicians at Virginia Mason to identify many different status quo approaches to work as highly wasteful and not patient focused. It was this approach to transparency and waste elimination that set the stage for the work described in this chapter.

## Breakthrough at Virginia Mason

The innovative breakthrough that Dr. Robert Mecklenburg and his colleagues at Virginia Mason Medical Center achieved started with a crisis. Mecklenburg was chief of medicine at Virginia Mason in 2004 when the insurance company Aetna threatened to exclude Mecklenburg's health care organization from an elite network. Aetna was in a powerful position as a purchaser of care for such major companies in the Greater Seattle area as Starbucks, Costco, and Alaska Airlines, among others. Losing this business would be a blow not only to Virginia Mason's finances but to the medical center's considerable prestige as well.

Aetna was not doing this on a whim. Aetna's data had revealed that Virginia Mason was more expensive than its major competitors in a number of important specialties. Mecklenburg and his colleagues were alarmed, although the more Mecklenburg thought about it the more he viewed the situation as a potential opportunity. He was deeply engaged in Virginia Mason's adaptation of the Toyota Production System as its management method and was working closely with Gary Kaplan and the rest of the Virginia Mason leadership team in that process. Kaplan, Mecklenburg, and their colleagues were in their fourth year of establishing the Virginia Mason Production System, and even though they had made great strides toward improving quality and controlling cost, they knew there was still a difficult road ahead. For one thing, Kaplan was receiving vigorous and often hostile pushback from many people within Virginia Mason, most notably a number of physicians. The idea that a car-manufacturing methodology could in any way apply to health care seemed ludicrous to them. But Kaplan could clearly see its application, and he pressed on with the active support and engagement of leading clinicians such as Mecklenburg.

During a series of discussions with Aetna and a conversation with benefits managers from a number of the major companies that were Aetna customers, Mecklenburg began to focus intently on the question of who his customer was. At Virginia Mason the patient was at the top of a pyramid that embodied the medical center's strategic plan and its vision to transform health care. But the fact was that employers paid the bills—paid huge dollars for their employees' care. Mecklenburg realized that neither he nor his physician colleagues had ever really considered the companies paying the bills as customers. In fact, Mecklenburg wasn't sure he or any of his colleagues had ever met with or talked to the people writing the checks.

Mecklenburg reflected on this and realized that all these major companies purchased services and materials from a wide variety of suppliers. He could see that Virginia Mason was one of those suppliers; a supplier in fact that provided a critically important and increasingly expensive set of services to employees. Health care costs were typically one of the leading employer expenses and the great majority of these companies managed their suppliers with rigor and discipline—with the notable exception of health care suppliers.

To gain a better understanding of what the employers wanted from him, Mecklenburg paid a visit to Annette King, the benefits manager for Starbucks, which is headquartered in Seattle. King was taken aback for she had never before had a doctor come to her office and ask her how he could improve care for her employees. Mecklenburg and King had an amiable discussion, which wound up centering on the problem of back pain among Starbucks workers. King said it was a significant problem for her workforce, causing pain and missed work and driving up her costs while hurting productivity.

Mecklenburg was genuinely surprised that large numbers of Starbucks workers suffered from back pain and that it had such a significant negative impact on the company. He left King's office with a sense of excitement. He had been working to adapt the Toyota principles and methods to the medical center's work and now he saw an opportunity to take those methods outside into the marketplace. It was, thought Mecklenburg, a huge opportunity, and Gary Kaplan saw it as "a call to arms." "It was the catalytic event we needed to develop clinical value streams," Kaplan says. "We were focused on the fact that we needed to understand the data and make the care better for the people who receive care, our patients, and more affordable for those who purchase care, their employers."

After a series of internal discussions Mecklenburg invited Starbucks and Aetna to join with Virginia Mason in forming what he called a *marketplace collaborative* to identify and solve the quality and cost issues around treatment of routine or uncomplicated back pain. Starbucks and Aetna agreed immediately and began working side by side with Mecklenburg and his team, including Dr. Andrew Friedman, head of the Virginia Mason spine clinic. After a series of discussions the collaborative settled on five principles. They agreed to

1. focus on customers' highest costs;
2. adopt customers' definition of quality;
3. create evidence-based clinical value streams;
4. employ systems engineering tools to remove waste;
5. use a cost reduction business model.

Friedman and his team had discovered that about 80 to 85 percent of patients with back pain suffer from an uncomplicated medical condition best cured by physical therapy; the remaining patients needed more advanced treatment. The collaborative identified uncomplicated back pain as a target of opportunity for improving efficiency and effectiveness in the delivery of care.

## The First Breakthrough Collaborative

At this point the Virginia Mason Production System began to play a defining role. Mecklenburg and his colleagues developed a value stream map of back pain care at Virginia Mason. This map defined each step in the process and revealed the current state of care—the reality. Kaplan referred to it as "draining the swamp" to see what was underneath. And what was underneath was distressing. The process was chaotic, immensely wasteful, not at all effective for patients—and needless to say, expensive.

The value stream map revealed that patients entered the spine clinic through various portals—via a primary care physician or specialist in neurology or neurosurgery. These visits, especially those with specialists, were extremely expensive and did very little if anything to help a patient with uncomplicated low back pain. Waits for appointments to see such specialists could run into months. Andrew Freidman commented that patients might have an MRI and "then have another wait to review that scan, then they would have another wait in order to finally get into physical therapy."

After carefully studying the value stream map, Mecklenburg told Annette King and other company representatives in the marketplace collaborative something none of them had ever heard from a physician before, something truly startling: "The value stream showed that most of our care process was no help at all," says Mecklenburg. The potential gains with the uncomplicated back pain patients was obvious: many were receiving MRI tests, for example, at a cost of $1,200 each to Starbucks, yet the evidence indicated that an MRI for patients with uncomplicated back pain provided zero clinical value. Needless waits and delays for care were substantial and did not add value. It was pure waste.

The collaborative members then focused on what King wanted for her employees, and they defined quality care—*from the customer's perspective*—as having five components:

1. Evidence-based care
2. 100 percent patient satisfaction
3. Same-day access
4. Rapid return to function
5. Affordable cost for both providers and employers

These elements guided Mecklenburg, Friedman, and their colleagues in radically reshaping Virginia Mason's treatment path for uncomplicated back pain. They started with a patient's initial call with a complaint of back pain. The team designed a standard series of evidence-based questions that separated patients with uncomplicated back pain from those needing emergent or complicated care. Those in the uncomplicated category would not wait. They would be seen that day—the same day they called. Patients would arrive and meet with a physical therapist (PT) for a fifteen-minute discussion of their condition. For an additional fifteen minutes a physician would join in and, sitting side by side with the PT, discuss the case and approve the treatment program. Patients would then have their first sixty-minute PT treatment.

This marketplace collaborative with Starbucks and Aetna could hardly have been more successful. After just ninety days, the new pathway had cut patients' waiting time for an appointment from an average of thirty-one days to same-day access. On top of that, the first year's data showed that 94 percent of patients were returned to work that day or the next. No prescription medications were needed in three-quarters of the cases, and patient satisfaction ratings were through the roof. The results were huge positives for the patients, for Starbucks, and for Aetna. And Virginia Mason turned its loss of revenue from unnecessary procedures (including unnecessary imaging tests) into additional capacity so that staff could see and treat many more patients.

## More Breakthrough Collaboratives

Mecklenburg and his colleagues established comparable marketplace collaboratives with various other companies in order to improve treatment for migraine headaches; breast nodules; shoulder, knee, and hip pain; acid reflux; and cardiac disease. Every collaborative achieved substantial improvement in value for purchasers and patients.

The Virginia Mason team also began a marketplace collaborative on imaging with the state of Washington purchasing arm, the Health Care Authority. This collaborative took the process Virginia Mason already had for determining whether back pain and headaches required imaging and added a similar process for sinus imaging, with the result that about 25 percent of advanced imaging studies in these three high-volume areas were eliminated. The dramatic reduction in the use of MRIs was an important finding that Mecklenburg and his colleagues shared with the broader medical community in the *Journal of the American College of Radiology* (Blackmore, Mecklenburg, & Kaplan, 2011).

The collaborative solution was simpler, more effective, and much more efficient than methods previously reported in the medical literature for reducing unnecessary imaging. The breakthrough feature was *mistake proofing*, a method learned from Toyota. A provider seeking to order an MRI of the lower back, for example, was presented with a series of checkboxes on the computer screen. Each box represented an evidence-based indication for the test. The test was scheduled when the patient checked a box, indicating an evidence-based reason for the test. One click of the cursor both scheduled the test and ensured that imaging was evidence based. If the patient showed none of the evidence-based indicators, the test could not be ordered. This method immediately and dramatically reduced utilization of advanced imaging. Just as important, it eliminated the need for costly commercial systems that require either time-consuming preauthorization or retrospective audits, reports, delays in payment, or lengthy appeal cycles. These costs are initially absorbed by providers but quickly shifted to employers through increased prices. Other provider groups in the Seattle market have replicated this method with similar success, and the Virginia Mason team offers the method free to anyone who wishes to use it.

## Spreading the Marketplace Collaborative Concept

Virginia Mason's singular success in adapting the Toyota Production System to health care resulted in a good deal of international attention. A steady stream of providers from around the world have traveled to Seattle to learn from Virginia Mason. To accommodate the growing demand, Kaplan founded the Virginia Mason Institute to share the organization's knowledge.

Similarly, the marketplace collaboratives were so successful that in 2007, Kaplan, Mecklenburg, and several colleagues founded the Center for Health Care Solutions at Virginia Mason Medical Center. It was among the most tangible efforts by the organization to pursue its commitment to transform health care, and Mecklenburg transitioned from chief of medicine to medical director of the new center. Mecklenburg was convinced that the marketplace collaborative model could be adopted anywhere in the United States and that it could have a significant impact on the health care quality and cost challenges facing the country. He believed it would improve access to care, as well. Although Mecklenburg liked much of what was contained in the Affordable Care Act of 2010, he worried that it would not provide enough help fast enough to companies struggling with the mounting costs of care for their employees. "The fundamental system is dysfunctional and the legislation does little in the short term to change that," he said not long after the law was enacted. In fact, he said, millions of new people would be brought into this existing wasteful system.

As he focused his work on the role of employers in improving cost and quality, Mecklenburg worried that without significant changes, the same trends that had existed for some years would continue and that employers would continue to shift the financial burden of unaffordable health care to their employees. This cost shifting could become a vicious cycle in which employees, who are even less able than employers to cope with the climbing cost of coverage, could end up in a terribly vulnerable position.

That there was no significant short-term relief for employers was where the real opportunity lay in Mecklenburg's view. The key to fostering rapid change and improvement in both quality and cost was through leveraging the purchasing power of employers. "Purchasing power can bring out the best in health care," he says, because if leveraged properly, it would improve quality, drive down cost, and create greater opportunities for access.

The lesson of these collaboratives was clear, says Mecklenburg. What we need from providers is the ability to produce quality health care. When providers eliminate waste and produce reliable, quality care, the cost declines. But health plans also have an essential role. They must align reimbursement with value, paying for "high quality and rapid access not poor quality, waits, and delays." He argues that if health plans continue to be willing to pay for poor-quality care, the marketplace will continue to produce poor-quality care. But if employers and public agencies purchase high-quality care, inefficient and ineffective care will be driven from the marketplace.

## Produce Quality; Pay for Quality; Purchase Quality

A fundamental problem, as Mecklenburg sees it, is that employers have been outsourcing the purchase of one of the most important inputs to their organizations: health care. And they have entrusted this most important responsibility to health plans that often have no economic incentive to purchase high quality care for employers. He argues that health plans too often do not purchase care efficiently or intelligently for their clients. In a better system, he says, "the job of health plans is simply to pay for quality. That is all they should do."

But because health plans do not do that, Mecklenburg believes that the solution is to have employers step in and do it themselves—or to use their leverage to make sure health plans do it. "Employers should take an active role themselves," he says. "*They should know what quality is and buy it.*" The difficulty, he says, is that the vast majority of employers do not shop prudently for themselves or their employees, nor do they recognize the difference between high-quality and poor-quality care. Employees end up with inconsistent, expensive health care and the employer—with a combination of employee and company money—picks up the tab.

Gary Kaplan often notes that the entire process would be helped if cost and quality metrics in health care were much more transparent than they currently are.

Mecklenburg's core belief, and the idea behind the marketplace collaboratives, is that "if you can define and measure quality, why don't you procure it with the care that you buy other goods and services? It is quite possible to define, measure, and report quality indicators for health care. What health care reform needs are employers willing to demand the best from providers and health plans for their employees."

## Intel Looks to Health Care to Improve Cost and Quality

Bob Mecklenburg and Pat McDonald had never met before September 18, 2007. They had traveled radically different professional pathways. Mecklenburg was a physician in a large medical center and McDonald was a plant manager for Intel, one of the world's leading technology companies and the largest semiconductor chipmaker ever. Pat's beginnings there were modest: she had started as a summer intern on the manufacturing floor in 1985 and by 2007 had worked her way up to become manager of Fab (fabrication plant) 20, then Intel's highest-performing chip factory in the world. Yet these very differences—combined with their mutual passion for improvement—would soon make Mecklenburg and McDonald one of the more innovative teams in American health care.

When they first met, McDonald and several of her Intel associates were visiting Seattle to attend a conference where Mecklenburg was one of half a dozen Virginia Mason people who presented that day. As part of the conference, a tour of Virginia Mason was offered, and McDonald and her team eagerly signed on. At Intel, getting inside a plant for a tour is all but impossible, so she jumped at the chance to see the Virginia Mason operations. She was intrigued by the whole concept of applying *lean* thinking and methods in health care and was eager to see exactly what that meant in reality.

The plan was to tour both the pediatric and sports medicine clinics, and when the group was led into pediatrics, McDonald recalled, "the biggest thing that hit me was there was no one in the waiting room. I thought, well, it's either staged or everyone is on break." But the reality was that the flow of work in pediatrics had been completely redesigned by teams of parents and providers—all the providers involved in pediatric care. The result was that patients were being seen within ten minutes of arriving at the clinic.

As a parent McDonald was impressed that "you don't have all the children in the waiting room coughing and crawling all over you. If you were there with a well child, you're not going to get a sick child right with him." She could also see that all supplies were in the exam rooms so that the care team did not have to go looking for anything. "It was clear they had the right tools at the right time at the right places, so it was very analogous to what you do on a manufacturing floor. On the other side—behind the curtain in the working area—they had a great monitoring system for the care units, and the provider teams were sitting together, which facilitates teamwork and communication. You could see engagement and facilitation of communication, and it was clear how that would lead to error proofing care of the patient."

McDonald was similarly impressed with the sports medicine section, where a physician on the tour asked a question of a Virginia Mason staff member. He said it was fine to see improvements in flow coming from lean methodology, but he wondered how or whether lean techniques had been used in clinical care.

The answer was absolutely—Toyota techniques had been applied throughout the clinical processes. For example, explained an RN, physicians and physical therapists at Virginia Mason had recognized that treatment of rotator cuff injuries varied widely, which meant not all patients were getting the best care. The clinical team worked together to identify and standardize a best practice for such injuries, and patients subsequently received that standard, best-practice care every time—no matter the provider.

When she left Virginia Mason to return to Portland, McDonald thought very seriously about her own work. She had attended a five-day lean training program in Detroit a couple of months earlier and come away not entirely sure how lean approaches would apply to her business. But seeing the applications in health care—given its immense complexity—impressed her. She realized that although she had applied some lean approaches in her factory, she had done so only in certain areas. And she had not applied the techniques in attempting to solve her most challenging and complex business problems. As she traveled back to Portland, she says, "my light bulb turned on and I thought, if Virginia Mason can apply lean methodology to health care, where peoples' lives and quality of life are at stake, I certainly can go back and apply it to the most complex problems in my factory."

But this would not be easy. McDonald's factory was recognized as a worldwide quality leader, and her manager told her, "Your biggest disadvantage in implementing lean is your success." Ironic of course but true in a way. Why mess with success?

But McDonald had a very good reason for wanting to bring lean tools and techniques to the factory: She was determined to achieve the ideal state—zero defects and zero quality events (at Intel, *quality events* were incidents that caused a disruption in normal manufacturing operations). She had reached an elite level of achievement through traditional management methods, but she believed that to push through to that ideal space, she needed something more rigorous; a method that would lay bare the manufacturing process and in so doing reveal any heretofore hidden glitches. She also believed that lean management would eliminate waste and make her operation even more efficient.

McDonald and her team intensified their efforts, developing tools and processes for delivering rapid, lean improvements in three-week cycles. Essentially, the team would identify an issue or challenge, examine it as a value stream, and determine what constituted a waste or delay and what constituted value. The team then worked to eliminate the waste and delays and focus only on what was value-added.

And it worked well in a number of areas. When her team had become more amenable to the lean methods, she decided it was time to tackle the toughest problem she faced. The unpredictable and recurring nightmares in her professional life were the rare but deeply troubling quality events in manufacturing. These somewhat silent and often hidden problems were by no means unique to Intel. In fact, they are inherent in technology manufacturing. The most troublesome aspect was that when a quality event occurred it might not be recognized at the time and could remain undetected until later—sometimes much later—in the manufacturing process. Quality events could be so serious that the production line would have to be slowed or even shut down altogether while the problem was resolved. Intel engineers could solve these problems once discovered, but McDonald and her team were determined to do better—to find them much earlier in the process, before they had a chance to cause an interruption in the manufacturing operations.

The deeper McDonald and her team dove into the problem using rapid lean tools—including direct observation and value stream mapping—the more they discovered parts of the engineering processes where standardization provided compelling improvements. Identifying and eliminating variation enabled the team to detect and fix problems more quickly, which improved the quality of products and controlled the cost of production.

The initial work focused on a part of the manufacturing process known as lithography. It would be difficult to overstate the significance of lithography—the process of printing a pattern on silicon wafers—in the manufacture of semiconductor chips. "Lithography is the heart and the most complex operation in semiconductor processing," says McDonald. "And the setup must be precisely correct." Controlling this operation is the daily work of the sophisticated engineering organization in a semiconductor manufacturing facility. Variation is the enemy. If McDonald and her team could identify variation during the manufacturing process rather than further downstream, it would enable them to make quick, cost-effective corrections.

They learned through the lean process that part of the problem was human variability, specifically variation among engineers. "We had not tackled the variation in decision making among the engineers because they were the experts, many of them doing it for decades," McDonald says. "And remember the backdrop—this was the highest-quality, lowest-cost factory. And you're telling the expert he's not doing his job?"

At one point McDonald thought the lean work had solved the issue, but soon afterward a quality event occurred. "We're thinking, 'life is good,' and then we hit a speed bump. We had a repeat quality event in a place we did not standardize," says McDonald. With the rapid lean tools in place, they "found it fast and fixed it fast." They succeeded in standardizing both the process and decision making. The improvements were a breakthrough. In less than a year McDonald and her team achieved their ideal state of zero quality events in the lithography process. The result of this work was not only a dramatic improvement in the manufacturing process but a new-found respect for the lean process generally and, in particular, for the work being done at Virginia Mason.

When he later heard about the work at Intel from Pat McDonald, Bob Mecklenburg was delighted it had gone so well and that the inspiration of Virginia Mason had played a small part. He also found it richly ironic. "The amazing thing to me was that a high-tech, high-performing manufacturing company like Intel would learn anything from Virginia Mason in terms of systems engineering," he says. "The further irony is that we had spent years translating our approaches from Japanese manufacturing to U.S. clinical care and then [making a] further translation from the language of clinical care to that of purchasers of health care. And here we were translating back again from the language of health care purchasers to that of clinical care to that of manufacturing. It struck me as unusual and remarkable and reinforced the thought that we were all converging on similar approaches for tackling the same fundamental problems."

## The Right Way to Do This Is to Put the Purchaser in Charge

As a plant manager Pat McDonald held one of the most challenging and critical roles within Intel Corporation. Part of succeeding at Intel meant managing and partnering with suppliers, and McDonald had done so through the years. She had also been successful at controlling costs in a wide variety of areas affecting manufacturing. But she had never given much thought to the cost of health care for Intel employees. That changed in 2009 when she was asked to join a committee—known at Intel as a *corporate strategic discussion*—to explore ways to control the rapidly rising costs of health care for Intel employees. "Health care was the only area of our business where we did not control quality and cost," she says. "And costs were out of control. When we manage equipment suppliers, we measure safety, quality, and cost. We weren't doing that with health care suppliers."

To say that Intel managed suppliers with discipline and rigor was to understate the reality by an order of magnitude. Intel's Supplier Continuous Quality Improvement (SCQI) Program "is an organized proven program for achieving extraordinary supplier performance," according to the company. "Suppliers continuously improve their products and services provided to Intel. The program rewards suppliers for quality results and behaviors." The company's Quality of Service Health Assessment "is used to assess a supplier's quality systems against a preestablished set of scoring criteria to determine if systems exist, effectiveness of the systems, and which areas need attention" (Intel Corporation, n.d.[a]).

These and a variety of other programs manage and refine the supplier process at Intel, using rigorous management and state-of-the-art technology. Yet the committee on which

McDonald was serving could see that similar rigor did not apply in health care.

The committee was fairly large, with twenty-plus members from many different areas of the corporation. The idea was to explore the whole topic of health and wellness and to ask how the company could deliver better services to employees while reducing costs. Committee members spent months listening to guest presentations from experts and reading many case studies. Finally, the group was convened for a discussion about what to do. Richard Taylor, an Intel vice president and director of human resources, led the session and asked each person in turn to make a recommendation. It so happened that Pat McDonald was the last to speak.

"If this problem was in manufacturing, the way we would approach it is we would apply lean," she said. One of the previous speakers had alluded to Virginia Mason's work with Boeing in Seattle, and McDonald remarked on that and added, "I have seen Virginia Mason and they have started working with employers, so why don't we apply lean to health care and see if we can copy what they are doing and reproduce it here?"

Richard Taylor liked the idea and gave McDonald the go-ahead to proceed along that pathway. She subsequently took the corporate strategic discussion group to Seattle to see Virginia Mason and, she says, to show the group "why I believed in their approach to apply lean to health care and the health care marketplace collaboratives. My point was that we could do that in Portland."

McDonald's Intel team included two senior lean practitioners, and HR executives, including Richard Taylor, who was also the executive sponsor of the project. The team also included a person from the Intel Digital Health Group, a joint venture with GE to develop services that help people live healthy, independent lives at home. In all, the team numbered around eight, and they spent the better part of a day at Virginia Mason. "We were expecting a slide show with one or two presenters not a whole fleet of doctors and nurses taking the time to tour us through Virginia Mason," says McDonald. "They gave us free, open, flowing dialogue—open access. It was amazing. Their openness and transparency was very impressive."

McDonald and her Intel associates also vividly recalled meeting Mecklenburg when they had visited two years earlier.

McDonald says that his professional standing and knowledge coupled with his striking sense of transparency had made for a powerful presentation. Mecklenburg had talked about his work and also about the Virginia Mason Production System and their effort to reach zero defects. He had acknowledged that Virginia Mason was not there yet and told a riveting and tragic story about a patient of his—Mrs. Mary McClinton—who had been given an intravascular injection of a colorless antiseptic that had been mistaken for an intended injection that was also colorless. The antiseptic injection was deadly, triggering a fatal shutdown of Mrs. McClinton's internal systems until she died, weeks later. The Intel team was struck by the fact that the Virginia Mason leadership had released the news publicly so that an understanding of this mistake—and the corrective actions that followed to prevent its recurrence—might help other provider organizations prevent a similar mistake. To the Intel team Mecklenburg had demonstrated not only a commitment to excellence but courage as well, and they felt a real sense of confidence in his professionalism.

Now, on their current visit, McDonald and her colleagues were also impressed with a tour of the Virginia Mason oncology unit, which had been thoroughly redesigned applying the principles and tools of the Toyota Production System. "They showed the redesign to get all oncology services on one floor," says McDonald.

> You could see that people were not just waiting around in a crowded room almost sitting on top of each other. They had a pleasant soothing spacious area. In the treatment rooms you could see how everything was brought to the point of service—to the patient. It was very serene, not rushed, not hurried. They talked about the immense change it took to get all docs and nurses to agree how to lay out oncology floor—to get the treatment at the point of activity and provide the right care at the right time.

> We saw where they did real-time blood work, and to us as engineers, seeing the rigor with which they were doing real-time

blood work—seeing incredible reductions in throughput times in terms of turning around the results to patients waiting to hear their latest results in their battle for life—it was quite impressive.

In one conference room, the Virginia Mason team had displayed a list of precisely what they had been working on with measurements indicating progress or lack of it. "It was an entire wall of key indicators," McDonald recalls, "exactly what they were working on in terms of continuous improvement and care delivery. And even to us as laypeople it was very clear the progress they were making."

When leaders at Virginia Mason talked about the Virginia Mason Production System they emphasized the specific work they had done around safety, quality, and cost, and McDonald was hearing "many of the same specifics we talk about at Intel when we talk about manufacturing." The Intel team was also struck by the openness displayed by Mecklenburg and the rest of the Virginia Mason presenters. They talked openly of challenges and barriers and in no way tried to sell any notion that their method was not without its imperfections or challenges. When Mecklenburg displayed the pyramid, a graphic representation of Virginia Mason's strategic plan, an ever-present guide for decision making with the patient at the top, it was clearly similar to the Intel approach of identifying the customer as their top priority.

Mecklenburg's message could hardly have been more direct: companies such as Intel should use their purchasing power to get the health care they deserved and were paying for. He compared the cost of care in the United States with the cost in other industrialized nations and said emphatically that Intel "should not be paying 40 percent more than [its] global competitors."

"We had hours together and we talked in detail about the barriers to health care reform," says Mecklenburg. "We talked about the challenges of producing quality and reimbursing for quality and purchasing quality." He talked in some detail about his experience with the Seattle marketplace collaboratives and what he had learned from that experience, that the collaborative was a practical model for harnessing the purchasing power of employers. He recounted some of the difficulties he had encountered along the way and expressed his strongly held conviction that "the right way to do this would be to put the purchaser in charge."

"It felt like we didn't have to do a whole lot of explaining to them," says Mecklenburg. "They quickly understood what we were talking about. The conversation flowed easily and was relaxed. They really understood what we were trying to do because they had been walking through the briar patch. What we were about was aspiring to produce the same value and pace of improvement they had demonstrated."

And Mecklenburg went on to mention the prediction of Intel cofounder Gordon Moore that "the number of transistors incorporated in a chip will approximately double every 24 months." As Intel has pointed out, "This forecast of the pace of silicon technology, popularly known as Moore's Law, was more than just a prediction. Essentially, it described the basic business model for the semiconductor industry. For more than four decades, Intel has delivered the challenge of Moore's Law" (Intel Corporation). Of course in health care, achieving an equivalent to Moore's Law is more complicated. Atul Gawande has noted that a physician with a new patient faces something on the order of 13,600 diagnostic options and over 6,000 medications to choose from. He has also observed that in the mid-1970s, a patient in a hospital required 2.5 staff FTEs (full-time equivalents) for their care and twenty years later, in the mid-1990s, the requirement was more than 15 (personal communication with Maureen Bisognano, 2011).

## Transferring Lean Lessons from Health Care to Manufacturing

On May 1, 2009, a few days after the Virginia Mason visit, Pat McDonald and the rest of the Intel team gathered back in Portland for a follow-up discussion. The group members discussed things they had seen and learned at Virginia Mason that they thought might apply to their situation at Intel. Their foundational question—whether Virginia Mason was for real—had been answered. The Intel team came away with no doubt that it was not only for real but that its people had achieved a high level of excellence in applying lean throughout the organization.

The team went through a process often used at Intel, with several steps including a discussion in which team members answer the question, "What did you see?"

They saw, for example, "cases of moving from doctor as customer to patient as customer." They saw a team that had overcome the "hierarchical structure of the medical industry" and turned it into a "collaborative team structure." They saw a top-down commitment from executives and the former chief of medicine (Mecklenburg) as well as "bottom-up ideas percolating at the grass roots." The Intel team saw empty waiting rooms in a service where the exam rooms were full; collaboration with business partners; a culture in which people were willing to take risks to improve care for patients. "We saw that they were the real deal," says McDonald. "We saw that they were advanced lean practitioners. We walked away believers. These folks genuinely know what they are doing and they were willing to share and be transparent in their practices. They were for real."

So much so that McDonald wanted to replicate the Virginia Mason marketplace collaborative model in Portland. The Intel team members liked the collaborative's experience of paying for value, and they were attracted to the way the companies in Seattle had engaged with the health care providers directly rather than working through the insurer. They were also attracted by the idea that the Virginia Mason experiments had informed and empowered patients. Their notes from the meeting convey their thinking clearly: The Intel team liked the "shared savings approach vs. winner/loser (specialist time focused on right patient, practicing their specialty—right patient, right time, right provider)." The idea that the Seattle marketplace collaboratives had succeeded in eliminating expensive, unnecessary treatments—MRIs, for example—while at the same time getting people back to work at peak efficiency very quickly was, of course, immensely appealing to Intel, for this was where the company's bottom line could be significantly improved.

McDonald could clearly see that Intel did not have the needed expertise in this area but that Mecklenburg was a technical expert with enormous experience and thus the ideal partner and adviser in the venture. As her notes indicated when the Intel team met back in Portland, "Dr. Mecklenburg is the expert/

coach for marketplace collaboratives." She also recognized a fundamental difference between what had happened in Seattle and what the team was thinking about for Intel. In Portland the marketplace collaborative would be led by Intel—an employer—not by a provider organization as had been the case in Seattle. This was no mere subtle difference. This in fact was what Mecklenburg urgently wanted—this was Virginia Mason's vision for where U.S. health care could go to improve quality and reduce cost: have employers exercise their market power and leverage to *purchase high-quality care and only high-quality care.*

"It is important that the collaborative be driven by an employer and not a provider or a health plan," Mecklenburg says. One main reason for this is that the motives of both providers and health plans are often suspect. "When a provider drives a marketplace collaborative, it does not have as much credibility as when an employer drives the collaborative. Providers have not always done their best for purchasers." Moreover, "a provider or health plan driving a collaborative oriented toward better, faster, more affordable [care] will likely not be as effective as when the actual purchaser—the stakeholder accountable for the health and well-being of employees—does it. The employer has a strong incentive to secure rapid, high-quality care to ensure a healthy, productive workforce to compete in the global marketplace. The employer has an immense stake in the good health of its employees."

With the employer driving the process it quickly becomes clear who is paying the bills, who has the purchasing power. It becomes obvious that both providers and health plans are employed by employers; that employers are paying the salaries of providers and health plan staff. In the marketplace collaboratives on which he worked in Seattle, Mecklenburg found that "it was often a challenge to get the employers to flex their muscles and use their purchasing power; to not be unduly influenced by the health plans and the doctors. Employers often hesitate to hold either doctors or health plans accountable for delivering the best in quality and value."

On June 2, 2009, just weeks after the Intel team's visit to Virginia Mason, Mecklenburg and Diane Miller, executive director of the Virginia Mason Institute (VMI), accepted an invitation to travel to Portland to meet with McDonald and her team.

"They wanted to seriously explore establishing a partnership with VM [Virginia Mason] to create a marketplace collaborative in Portland—to copy exactly what VM had done in Seattle," says Mecklenburg. "This was a big deal. I thought it would be remarkable to line up these two organizations around health care. I had practiced for over thirty years and there weren't many things that would get my pulse rate up too much, but this was one of them: a defining moment." With Intel involved, Mecklenburg believed the business community throughout the country was likely to take notice and thereby increase employer demand for high-quality, high-value health care.

The message from McDonald to Mecklenburg and Miller was simple: We would like to copy exactly what you are doing. To do that, McDonald wanted to form a partnership with the Virginia Mason Institute whereby Mecklenburg would act as counselor and guide to Intel throughout the process. Before drawing up and agreeing on a contract, however, McDonald hosted a session in Portland where the Intel and Virginia Mason teams went through a process of identifying the *gives* and *gets* for each side.

The June 2 meeting brought together Bob Mecklenburg and Diane Miller from Virginia Mason with the Intel team of Pat McDonald, Kevin Carmody, Brian DeVore, Dr. Don Fisher, and Richard Taylor. The facilitators were Matt Brownfield and Wendy Fedderly, senior Intel lean management experts.

The objectives were clearly stated in the slide that kicked off the meeting:

- Form a collaborative team with Intel and VMI.
- Understand and agree to the value added proposition for Intel and VMI (note: *value added* is defined as what each will add, and what each is willing to pay for).
- Plan the process for Phase I partner selection, in a way that will positively disrupt the health care system in Portland, and get the attention of the largest providers in the Portland area.

The group identified the ideal state from Intel's point of view: to "pay for value" and to provide the right care in the right place at the right cost and the right time. The ideal state would include a focus on wellness and an "absence of need for reactive care due to flawless performance on proactive care." It would also be defined by the "elimination of errors: zero defects."

This approach, which had helped to guide the collaborative work at Virginia Mason, "really resonated with us," says McDonald. "The elimination of errors—zero defects—is language we use in our factories."

With Intel's aspiration for an ideal state defined, the question became how would the team try to achieve it? And the answer came in the form of a pyramid (Figure 2.1)—largely, though not entirely, copied from the pyramid that spells out Virginia Mason's principles and its vision "to be the Quality Leader and transform health care."

"We talked about our mutual goals," McDonald says, "what we each had to give to the formation of a market collaborative and what we would get out of working with each other."

## Figure 2.1.  Intel Guiding Principles

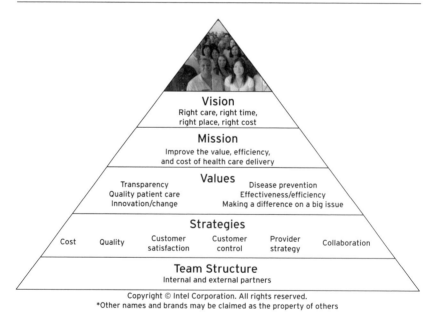

*Source:* Intel Corporation.

The gives and gets approach was familiar to the Virginia Mason team. Early on in his tenure as CEO in fact, Gary Kaplan and his leadership team had gone through a challenging process that led to agreement on a compact with the Virginia Mason physicians—essentially a gives and gets agreement between doctors and the organization. The Intel and Virginia Mason meeting was designed to identify areas of agreement and disagreement between the two organizations' teams, but as the meeting progressed it became clear that there were no areas of substantial disagreement and many areas where their interests aligned.

Intel would get superb clinical guidance from the developer of the marketplace collaborative concept, and Virginia Mason would get to test its work in a new market with one of the nation's blue-chip companies. Most important, if the collaborative was successful, Intel employees would get better quality care at a more affordable price. Or as McDonald put it, "the right care at the right time at the right cost."

From McDonald's perspective, Intel wanted to affiliate with a highly credible health care provider organization. "One of our internal values at Intel is technical expertise, and we were very conscious that we were not the technical experts in health care," she says. McDonald also emphasizes what a central role Mecklenburg played from the start. "He was really our voice of confidence—'you guys can do this,'" she says. "And he had proof of concept because he could talk about work the Virginia Mason team had already done. I don't think we really got the concept of using our purchasing power, because we were daunted by the fact that we were not the technical experts. But his message was, 'you are the employer. You are paying the bill. You need to sit down with providers and specify what you'll pay for.'"

Ultimately, of course, this made perfect sense to McDonald. "That's the way we handle our other suppliers," she says. Intel's manufacturing equipment suppliers were improving quality and reducing cost year after year, "but we were not taking the same approach in health care."

McDonald felt hopeful. She and her colleagues had worked well with Mecklenburg and Miller, and it was clear now to McDonald—clearer than it had been before—that the timing of the work was just right and that Mecklenburg was right when he said that as an employer Intel possessed significant market clout. "I've been in thousands of meetings and many are sort of vague; heads nod affirmation but when you finish the meeting it's not like there is strong agreement, it's often a more casual agreement," says Mecklenburg. "This is not the case with Intel. These are decisive people."

There was clear definition about what each side would contribute and get in return. Mecklenburg, for Virginia Mason, would provide content and counsel based on his experience with the Seattle marketplace collaboratives. He would help guide Intel in trying to copy what he had done in Seattle. Mecklenburg would review and analyze claims data to identify areas of heavy cost for Intel. He would advise providers what they could do to be successful within the collaborative.

In exchange, Intel's major give was that they were spreading the Virginia Mason concept to another major marketplace and they would compensate Virginia Mason for Mecklenburg's time and for the purchase of value stream maps Virginia Mason had completed for a variety of care areas including low back pain. Figures 2.2 and 2.3 display what the gives and gets from the meeting looked like after the session.

Though the Intel team was initially uncertain that the company had the market power to leverage providers, Mecklenburg continuously reassured them. "We found that [in 2008] 20 percent of all claimants drove 64 percent of all health care costs in Oregon," says McDonald. "That 5 percent drives 39 percent and the next 5 percent drives 12 percent."

McDonald aspired to spend 80 percent of Intel's health care dollars on prevention and wellness, leaving 20 percent or so to cover those who needed more intensive care and treatment. The company data were interesting for they showed that during 2008 and 2009, about 25 percent of the ailments suffered by Intel employees were musculoskeletal. But this 25 percent accounted for 55 percent of the company's health care cost. In addition, these ailments caused employees to miss work, thus increasing the cost to Intel. In a close examination of claims data from many employers, Mecklenburg found their major costs. First was the cost of screening and prevention that included office visits, blood work, and tests such as

**Figure 2.2. Intel Gives and VMI Gets**

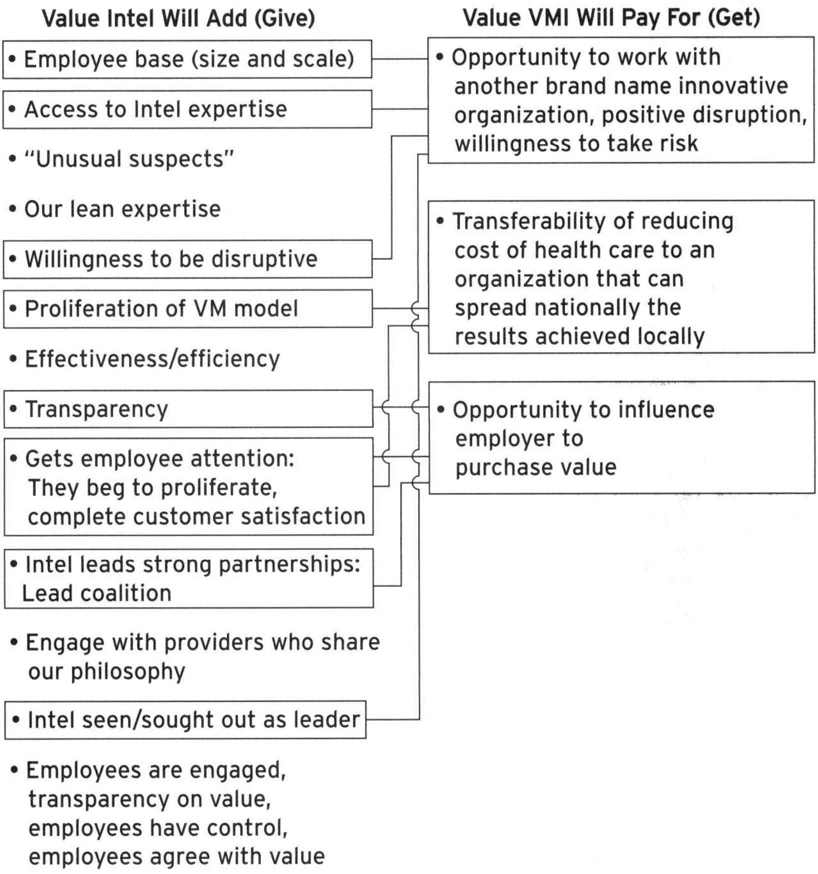

| Value Intel Will Add (Give) | Value VMI Will Pay For (Get) |
|---|---|
| • Employee base (size and scale) | • Opportunity to work with another brand name innovative organization, positive disruption, willingness to take risk |
| • Access to Intel expertise | |
| • "Unusual suspects" | |
| • Our lean expertise | • Transferability of reducing cost of health care to an organization that can spread nationally the results achieved locally |
| • Willingness to be disruptive | |
| • Proliferation of VM model | |
| • Effectiveness/efficiency | |
| • Transparency | • Opportunity to influence employer to purchase value |
| • Gets employee attention: They beg to proliferate, complete customer satisfaction | |
| • Intel leads strong partnerships: Lead coalition | |
| • Engage with providers who share our philosophy | |
| • Intel seen/sought out as leader | |
| • Employees are engaged, transparency on value, employees have control, employees agree with value | |

mammograms and colonoscopies. Next came upper respiratory ailments and then musculoskeletal issues, including back, knee, hip, and shoulder ailments.

The group could see that Providence Health & Services, a not-for-profit network of hospitals, health plans, and physicians, and Tuality Healthcare, a much smaller community-based provider in Portland, were logical choices for Intel's collaborative, as was CIGNA, one of the health plans serving Intel. Initially, there was some concern among the group members about

## Figure 2.3. VMI Gives and Intel Gets

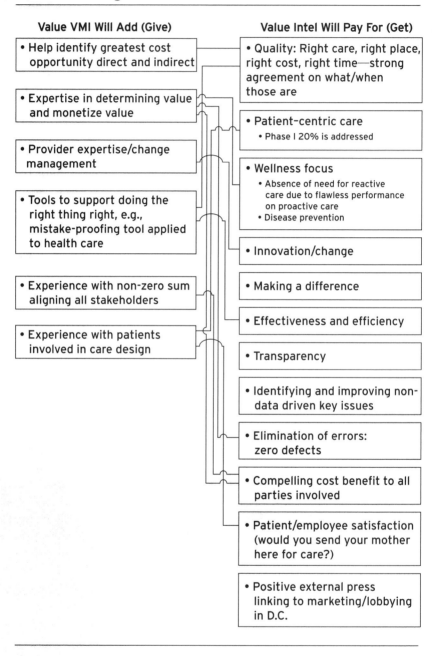

whether the doctors at Tuality and Providence would be willing to participate. Mecklenburg was amused by this.

"Can we really talk with these doctors?" McDonald asked Mecklenburg.

"I said, 'Pat, they will be here in ten minutes,'" recalls Mecklenburg. "It took almost zero effort to line up the providers. Intel is the customer every provider wants."

## Intel Uses Purchasing Power to Put the Patient First

On September 28, 2009, McDonald, joined by Mecklenburg, hosted a meeting of the collaborative participants at the Venetian Restaurant in Hillsboro, Oregon. About thirty-five people in all, from Intel, Providence, Tuality, and CIGNA, attended. McDonald talked about Mecklenburg's work in Seattle, and she explained that she wanted to get a better grasp on quality improvement and cost control for Intel employees. She also talked about the crucial role that lean principles played at Virginia Mason and at her Intel plant, citing the results of her lean work.

One of the most striking aspects of the meeting to McDonald was the unanimity among the providers about wanting to put the patient at the top of the pyramid. Gathered at the meeting were physicians, nurses, physical therapists, and administrators, and all were deeply committed to doing what was best for the patient. "They all share that higher level goal," says McDonald. "It's unique to their field. I had been involved in semiconductor consortiums for many years and there was no higher level goal that could tie everyone together. But here we were talking about something that was *for the good of a human being*. That's an amazingly powerful area of inclusion and it is very difficult for anyone to walk away from that."

The meeting was also a key moment for Mecklenburg, who witnessed the purchasing power of Intel. "Pat could see the power and influence she had as a purchaser," he says. "Pat felt her authority, her ability to help providers and health plans move in the right direction. She understood that she is the customer and these are her suppliers who will do what she wants and that was a wonderful moment—to see Pat gain confidence in this domain."

When Mecklenburg spoke at the session he sought to convince Providence, Tuality, and CIGNA that by changing the way they delivered certain care they had the chance to significantly improve quality and efficiency. He also sought to reassure providers "that this was going to be OK. That they weren't going to harm the finances of their institutions."

The fact that Mecklenburg had been a practicing physician for more than three decades as well as chief of medicine at Virginia Mason and a member of the Virginia Mason board of directors—in addition to his marketplace collaborative experience—gave him great credibility with the provider groups. Providers were hesitant, Mecklenburg says, to ask accountability of health plans, who control the flow of crucial information. The role of health plans is a particular sticking point for Mecklenburg, who is frustrated that health plans control essential information that both providers and employers need to improve the cost picture for employees. "Health plans control billing data and are in the position of using that data to interpret value for employers," he says.

> Billing data clearly conveys information about cost and this
> is very important, but billing data is not designed to measure
> quality or value and has serious limitations in these areas. For
> example, billing data cannot tell if an MRI is necessary or not, if
> it was interpreted correctly or if the care that followed the MRI
> was appropriate. Absence of billing data for a flu shot from a
> primary care provider does not mean that the patient did not
> obtain a free flu shot at work. Health plans are in a good position
> to be arbiters of cost but are not in a good position to be reliable
> arbiters of quality or value.

Mecklenburg is also concerned that providers have generally not been particularly skilled at gathering good data concerning the quality of care provided to their patients, and that providers have ceded this critical role to health plans. Thus, he says, "health plans become arbiters of quality by default."

In a marketplace collaborative, however, the employer and provider together define and measure quality. For marketplace collaboratives to be successful, they must have what Mecklenburg describes as *actionable information*: that is, data that reveal areas that can be targeted for quality and cost improvement. "What the health plan should contribute is actionable cost information based on all these millions of transactions, claims, that is organized in a way to help inform decisions," he says. But health plans do not typically package the data that way. "It does not come across as actionable information," he says. "It comes across as scrambled and unapproachable data. You have to find all the various line items that health plans use to process for billing for back pain entries in order to understand the real cost to the employer of uncomplicated back pain. When you start to use a little more sophisticated approach to analyzing the data, you can create actionable information from claims data. You can find the top ten conditions in terms of cost to the employer that are appropriate for reducing unnecessary cost. It then becomes apparent where opportunity is for providers and employers."

The first step for the Portland collaborative members needed to be training. The teams from Providence, Tuality, and CIGNA agreed to participate in a five-day lean methods class hosted by Intel just prior to Thanksgiving 2009. And it was during that week-long session that the participants in the collaborative began to find common ground. Although McDonald knew the training would establish a common language as well as lean tools for improvement, she had not anticipated that the two competing provider organizations would begin sharing right away, yet they did. "They have this overriding value and it is amazing to see these health care providers together," she says. "The thing that unifies them, that helps them transcend their position or organization, is their commitment to do things for the good of their fellow human beings."

## Making Care Better, Faster, and More Affordable

The Intel-driven Portland Healthcare Marketplace Collaborative was officially launched on December 1, 2009. The meeting room walls were plastered with data—current state and ideal state. McDonald emphasized lean work and Mecklenburg, delivering a sort of keynote, explained how he considered this a win-win for providers and employers.

He led the group through the value stream map for uncomplicated back pain, which revealed massive waste and focused the solution not with specialists but with physical therapists—the key to the success of the effort in Seattle. The room was jammed with representatives from the two provider organizations—Providence and Tuality—and although they were committed to the work, they were not without misgivings. There was concern expressed about losing money and about having unfilled appointments. How can you hold appointments open so that patients could have same-day access? What if the slots went unfilled? There was concern among the doctors about one of the big differences between this effort and the work in Seattle. At Virginia Mason the physicians are employees of the medical center whereas in Portland the doctors worked in independent groups. How could that be overcome?

At this point Mecklenburg took a step back, explaining that he believed that health care in the United States was unaffordable because the processes for paying for care, purchasing care, and delivering care had failed. The challenge for providers, he said, was to produce value-added care. He emphasized the high cost of imperfect quality, saying that the line items in claims data for complications—"imperfect quality"—"cost the employer twice what breast cancer and diabetes and depression cost" to treat and "four times what stroke and colon cancer cost." He estimated that "at least half of that is avoidable." He said that delays in access exacted high costs as well. "What does it cost to have someone off work?" he asked. "A three-day wait for an appointment may cost the employer more than an MRI, for example. That is why same-day access and rapid return to function is so important."

This all meant that change was necessary. A standardized systems approach would build in quality through evidence-based medicine and patient-centered care. It would build in speed, providing patients with just what was needed, when and where it was needed. The result would be less waste and lower cost; care that would be, in the words of the Mecklenburg mantra, "better, faster, more affordable."

He explained that the marketplace collaborative model would allow its participants to produce better, faster, more affordable care if three things happened: if employers used their purchasing power "to specify standards of quality, timeliness, and price"; if providers were to "produce value, improve [the] quality of health care, and increase access"; and if health plans were to "reduce costs to employers by rapidly aligning reimbursement with value." He explained that the Seattle marketplace collaboratives had demonstrated that customers—individuals and employers paying for care—needed these five dimensions of quality from providers: (1) evidence-based care, (2) 100 percent patient satisfaction, (3) same-day access, (4) rapid return to function, and (5) affordable cost for both providers and employers.

He showed a slide of the original Virginia Mason back pain value stream map that had revealed that nearly everything the medical center was doing was wasteful: that is, added no value. "I wanted to see the opportunities for improvement," he says. "I wanted to convey the humility that is the necessary first step for self-improvement. When you say that on a relative scale we're outstanding but on an absolute scale we're no good, it shows a great opportunity for improvement."

He then displayed the new value stream for care from the Seattle Marketplace collaborative, which showed an order of magnitude improvement on every measure. He offered metrics demonstrating that companies saved millions with the new approach, that patients got back to work much faster, that patient satisfaction was through the roof, and that provider finances not only survived the changes but thrived. "We showed that this model does not harm providers financially," he says. "Access is improved and throughput increased because they have a desirable product and there is a reduced cost of production because it requires *fewer* FTEs to deliver *more* care. Margin for providers increases as cost for employers decreases."

The substantive case for marketplace collaboratives was compelling if not overwhelming. But Mecklenburg also knew there was an issue that lay beyond the substantive, an issue or perhaps series of questions that troubled the doctors, in particular. And he did his best to address those questions during the session.

They had the same fears and concerns I had when we had started the process in Seattle at VM. I had lived through this. There had been a question about my identity as a physician when we began to create teams that used standardized process and a prominent role for nonphysician providers. When you talk about standard work and the increased value of physical therapists versus doctors, there is concern. "You mean I'm going to give up control of this patient to someone who doesn't have the knowledge or training I have?" "Is the PT going to be up to this?" "Am I still valuable as a physician?"

The toughest thing about being a doctor *by far* is the fear of harming people. I have awakened at 4:00 AM with "demons," worried about my care of a patient. Had I done everything right with Mrs. Jones in the ICU? Did I order the serum potassium, or was I distracted with other calls, pages, and the care of other patients? So I'd get up and call the ICU because I can't remember if I ordered the potassium level. This situation is typical of a system that depends on individual performance of physicians. Docs make an extraordinary effort to manage the dynamic environment of patient care as isolated individuals and without help from fail-safe systems, so it is no wonder that they have concerns that they can delegate their tasks to others.

We have this sacred trust and when we don't get it right we can kill people, so now we're saying to doctors that they should turn over the patient to someone less trained in a system we know is dysfunctional and we're still asking the doc to be accountable. "Is the PT going to miss important medical items I am accountable for? Will they miss a spinal tumor?" "What's my value to the system?" "Are they going to be able to do as good a job as I can?"

"And what does this do to my financing and kids' education and my mortgage payments?" "Is my salary going down?" These are concerns I had as an independent practitioner, as a section head, and as the chief of medicine. I knew these docs in Portland would be worried about this and I tried to reassure them that, of course, they are highly valuable, that the PT would do a good job because they were going to install fail-safe systems for the entire team, that they weren't going to lose salary, that they would have safe practices; that they would do a better job with more patients; and that this new approach would allow them to deliver more care and better quality care.

The Portland marketplace collaborative started with uncomplicated back pain because it was an ongoing problem for Intel employees and an expensive malady for the company, in terms of both direct cost of care and indirect cost—employees missing work or coming to work in pain. It was a good place to start because it was a fairly straightforward problem, and the value stream map that Virginia Mason had created in Seattle showed a clear pathway to a more efficient way to deliver care.

Perhaps most significantly, it was also a statement by Intel that the company had decided to use its purchasing power "to nudge providers toward standardization," as Mecklenburg put it. It was, of course, unusual in America for companies to get involved on the clinical side in an effort to improve care and control costs for its employees. But the inexorable and seemingly uncontrollable rise in health care costs from providers in recent years drove Intel to the point where it saw no alternative but to try to manage health care as it did other suppliers.

But nothing was automatic. Nothing was a given. McDonald and Mecklenburg had no intention of barging into the Portland medical community and throwing down a gauntlet. Certainly, however, Intel's marketplace clout was a major factor in its ability to quickly convene providers from both Providence health system and Tuality, a small community hospital in the geographical region where many Intel employees lived and worked.

Mecklenburg, in particular, was sensitive to not overstepping his bounds with medical colleagues in Portland. The physicians from Providence and Tuality were "well-qualified, highly experienced practitioners," he says.

> Dr. Tom Lorish from Prov is the local authority on this stuff. I'm not an authority on back pain. I had worked with authorities, including my colleague at Virginia Mason Dr. Andrew Friedman. And I had studied this a lot, but I had no direct credentials as a practitioner of musculoskeletal disease. Tom is a physiatrist, board certified in physiatry. The same with Dr. Mary K. O'Neil from CIGNA, a board certified physiatrist. I am coming to them with a different model of configuring care, and I'm going to try and reach common ground with experts in this condition. My task was to reach accord with these two content experts.

But the evidence for a different approach to treating uncomplicated low back pain in a different way was overwhelming—and not new to either Lorish or O'Neil. They had studied this area over the years, and they agreed that patients with uncomplicated low back pain received a lot more medical resources than were necessary or appropriate and that a new care pathway was needed.

"We all felt this was an area of improvement for the community and that it was particularly important for patients and employers and that we had an obligation to do better," says Mecklenburg. "Mary Kay and Tom are team-minded, community-minded practitioners. They had the capacity to embrace change and they did so. This is very important in terms of [the] change management piece of this. You need people who are confident and are unafraid of change, who are fundamentally unthreatened by change." And Lorish certainly fit that description. He had developed innovative programs for low back over the previous couple of decades, and he was attracted to Mecklenburg's approach because engaging with large employers meant obtaining a patient base large enough to make a specialized back program work.

## Mapping the Value Stream and Finding Improvements to VM's Process

Intel relied on a precise, two-step process to take on large, complex problems, and the Intel team applied this process with the collaborative. Step one involved *premapping*—identifying key elements of the solution—and *mapping* involved pulling all the many disparate elements of the execution plan together.

On December 17, 2009, participants in the collaboration gathered for a premapping session. This was a tried-and-true Intel practice in which McDonald had great confidence. "With large, complicated projects, if you get content experts together ahead of time, you can create a timeline divided into parallel work streams and then you have events and deliverables for each work stream," she says. "Premapping allows the content experts to start filling out the specific path in their area of expertise."

The premapping session ended with a determination of how ready participants were for mapping day, when the highly detailed plan for the back pain collaborative would be laid out. The Intel technique requires that participants indicate how strongly they agree with two specific questions: *what* the objective is, and *how* they will attain it. McDonald says that "when you ask, 'Do we all understand what we are trying to achieve and how we will achieve it?' usually people understand with 90-percent-plus clarity *what* we are trying to achieve, but very often on the *how* it's something like 50 percent. Then we ask, 'What would it take to get you to get closer to 100 percent on both?'"

In response to questions about the *how*, McDonald and Mecklenburg went back over the process Virginia Mason and others used in the Seattle marketplace collaboratives. "VM had developed and implemented it, and they shared their learning and they shared the fact that outcomes were predictable both clinically and financially," says McDonald. "It was clear to people we could learn from that value stream to implement and develop ours in Portland."

Map day was January 8, 2010. The participants—about 50 people in all from Intel, Providence, Tuality, and CIGNA—convened at a Courtyard Marriott to map out the existing state of treatment for uncomplicated low back pain. The large group was divided into smaller segments with each subgroup assigned a particular area of the low back pain treatment process to study and map out. When the participants arrived, all of the work for various swim lanes—a visual representation of the process steps—was already posted on the map. In all, it was about eight feet high and ran along two walls for more than thirty feet. The collaborators then proceeded to walk through the map, step-by-step, week-by-week, determining precisely what tasks had to be accomplished to implement the back pain value stream at Providence and Tuality.

When they began digging into specifics, they were faced with the five-dimension definition of quality that had been developed by the Seattle marketplace collaboratives and which Intel wanted adopted in Portland: (1) evidence-based care, (2) 100 percent patient satisfaction, (3) same-day access, (4) rapid return to function, and (5) affordable cost for both providers and employers. If this collaborative was going to work, the group as a whole had to approve all five dimensions of the model, and after some discussion they did so. However, in the course of this discussion it became clear that achieving these five dimensions would require a systems approach to providing care; a systems approach with rather strict control of variation in order to increase reliability. It would be an approach, as Mecklenburg put it, that was "systems dependent not operator dependent."

As much as the stars seemed to be aligned in Portland for precisely this type of approach, there remained unanswered questions. "One of the precarious, less-certain dimensions of health care reform on a larger scale," says Mecklenburg, "is whether a plan developed somewhere else will be acceptable and transferable to the providers, to a new health plan, a new employer, a new marketplace with perhaps a different culture."

In Seattle the Virginia Mason team had eliminated huge amounts of waste from the process of treating low back pain. Waiting time had gone from thirty-one days to same-day access. Wasteful employer spending on imaging tests and specialist appointments had been eliminated. The process had been trimmed down to just what the patient needed to get better and no more. At least that is what the team had believed. But in Portland Dr. Tom Lorish and others pushed to streamline the process even more, to make it even leaner and less costly while maintaining everything needed for quality. And the main change that Lorish suggested was eliminating the physician from the process. His basic case was that the access tool—the five screening questions asked over the telephone by the person scheduling the appointment and then reviewed a second time by the physical therapist—was sufficient and anything more was wasteful. He argued that the physician added no value.

Mecklenburg was a bit taken aback by this. Although he and his colleagues at Virginia Mason had discussed this possibility, they had decided to keep the doctor involved for that fifteen-minute segment when the physician and PT together met with the patient. But the Portland marketplace collaborative team wanted to push the process further and believed patients would be fine with seeing the PT only and not the doctor. In addition, Lorish noted that eliminating the doctor from the routine part of the process would make the job of scheduling patients into the clinic vastly easier. Instead of having to coordinate the schedules of physical therapists and doctors as was the case in Seattle, it would be a simple matter of slotting a patient in with the PT.

Mecklenburg was apprehensive. What happens, he said, if the access tool—the five screening questions designed to identify patients with uncomplicated back pain—somehow proved flawed or unreliable? What if patients were underestimating their symptoms? Or misrepresenting their symptoms? Mecklenburg had found in Seattle that between 5 and 10 percent of patients who had successfully gotten through the access tool actually had symptoms more challenging than the uncomplicated treatment stream could handle, and these patients were referred to other doctors for examination and treatment. "When the doctor is there with the patient embedded in the process this is less of a problem," says Mecklenburg. "The doctor is backing up the PT, retaking pertinent parts of the history. This is a conservative thing we did in Seattle for redundancy to back up the PT."

But was it *necessary*? Because if it was not necessary for the patient's well-being, it was waste. And that was how Lorish and others in Portland viewed it. Mecklenburg and his colleagues in Seattle had discussed the same issue themselves in some depth but had decided in the end to be conservative. Lorish had a different take on it. He had previously established a program at Providence in which core groups of physical therapists in various clinics focused on active treatment for low back pain. In this program, when patients called in they were scheduled to see the PTs without seeing a physician in the interim. Lorish found that in a typical case the patient dramatically improved after anywhere from two to six sessions with a PT. In cases where patients had more complex issues, the PTs referred them to doctors.

Having served as a member of the physical therapy board in Oregon, Lorish says he knew the PTs "could do initial evaluation and screening." Lorish also knew that open access was much more easily achieved in a PT clinic, which had the framework to take on a large patient caseload more quickly than a physician practice could. More than that, Lorish believes that when doctors treat uncomplicated low back pain they are operating at the lower end of their licenses, whereas when physical therapists treat it they are operating at the top of theirs. Given his experience and knowledge of how physical therapists worked, Lorish felt great confidence that the therapists would be able to manage the patients quite well without a doctor's intervention. And he noted that in Oregon, the law allowed patients direct access to physical therapists without a physician referral, which is not the case in many other states.

Mecklenburg was persuaded by Lorish's experience and reasoning, but he had one request, he says: "I asked that the doctor be available close by so that when you had one of these situations, . . . the physical therapist was not in a position of trying to convince a doctor to come across the street or [from] four blocks away, so that the doc was immediately available to see the patient."

Before a final decision was made on this issue the Portland collaborative members decided to try a three-month experiment. They set up processes for treating uncomplicated low back pain both at Providence and at Tuality, with everything being the same except that at Tuality doctors would be involved in precisely the same way doctors were at Virginia Mason and at Providence the doctors were not involved. "We proposed to try both models in parallel fashion to see if there was a difference," says Mecklenburg. "To see if patients had lower satisfaction rates without the doctor involved, to see if they recovered as quickly, to see if the physical therapists were anxious about not having a doc with them."

The experiment was not perfect because the numbers of patients involved during this period were small, but the bottom line was that there appeared to be no discernible difference between the two approaches. The Portland collaborative had improved on the value stream achieved in Seattle while retaining standardization and reliability.

Eventually, the Portland marketplace collaborative developed a new health care service for back pain, called DirectLine to Healthcare. It was initially offered only to Intel employees by both Providence and Tuality at their medical facilities, but a month later the service was offered to all patients at these providers. Instead of waiting days for an appointment, an individual using DirectLine to Healthcare meets with a medical provider within twenty-four hours of his or her phone call.

## Erasing a Gap in the Value Stream

The issue of whether or not doctors would be involved in the treatment process for uncomplicated low back pain was not the only hurdle the collaborative faced before the new service could be instituted. During the collaborative's value stream mapping process, each subgroup identified the activities related to its particular area. Each subgroup also had a leader or spokesperson who would stand in the middle of the room and walk along the map as he or she explained what the group proposed for the new process. The groups were thus able to identify redundancies, waste, and gaps. The product of this work was a highly detailed value stream map that showed each step in the process of a patient going through treatment at Tuality and Providence.

When they had completed the mapping process Pat McDonald looked at it and saw a huge gap. Many project activities were crammed into the time between January and April 1, 2010, and then there was a blank space until June 1, the date they had decided to launch the project and see the first patient. McDonald asked the group why the providers could not see their first patient on April 1. An intense debate ensued, with many reasons offered to explain why it was sensible and prudent to wait until June 1 and why April 1 would not work. But McDonald did not believe that. One enhancement developed in Intel's Rapid Integrated Lean process is *cadence*, a three-week cycle time for improvements. It was this approach McDonald had in mind as she urged the attendees to revise the schedule and to break the remaining work into three-week cycle times.

As the debate progressed, McDonald asked: "What's the right thing to do for the patient?"

And Janet Meyer from Tuality responded immediately, "You're right. We're forgetting who's at the top of the pyramid."

Every week thereafter the members of the collaborative's steering committee would meet to walk the map—literally walk along the map discussing tasks, challenges, deadlines, coordination, and more. "We walk the map every meeting," says McDonald. "What is the status on training, on communications, on finance, on clinical?"

McDonald and others leading the collaborative also invested time doing direct observation of work in the Providence and

Tuality clinics to determine the current state. The providers "allowed us to go into their clinics and directly observe the process from check-in until treatment, with the permission of the patient," she says. "What really impressed me was how caring and outgoing the physical therapists were in the patient's whole life, not just with their back pain. They would have personal conversations. Not just you're here; we need to get treatment done and send you on your way. These personal conversations allowed the physical therapists to learn more and more about the patient's habits, and they were able to give better coaching in terms of taking care of back and weight and smoking status."

In early February the physical therapists, who would be so crucial to the success of the uncomplicated back pain collaborative, were invited to Virginia Mason in Seattle to see the Virginia Mason back pain clinic in action.

## Launching the Treatment Program

Five weeks after the collaborative commenced, Pat McDonald provided a status update on the project to Steven Megli, her manager at Intel, vice president of the Technology and Manufacturing Group, and co-general manager of Assembly Test Manufacturing. Megli liked the collaborative's work enough that he authorized a budget to provide full-time employees to work on the collaborative at Intel. This was greatly helpful to McDonald, who at the time was moving to a bigger job within Intel, from plant manager at FAB 20 to director of the Product Health Enhancement Organization, which was designed to apply software programs to test Intel products for quality and reliability before shipping.

When the project commenced on April 1, it was overseen by a team led by McDonald that included providers from Tuality and Providence, personnel from CIGNA, and Bob Mecklenburg. The members of this core team met weekly—with some participants calling in if necessary—to review where the project stood and the work that needed to be done going forward.

On August 17, 2010, the Portland marketplace collaborative's effort focused on shoulders, knees, and hips was launched. The team members applied the lessons learned from their work on back pain to defining and mapping a process for treating uncomplicated shoulder, hip, and knee problems, and this new program was implemented on October 18, 2010. After just eight months these results were reported:

- Patient satisfaction 97 percent
- Same-day access 91 percent
- Rapid return to function 100 percent
- Use of evidence-based medicine 78 percent

The individual numbers are impressive but McDonald looks at the work from a broader standpoint. Considering the uncomplicated back pain treatment program, for example, she says that the cycle time for care was reduced from fifty-two to twenty-one days. "When you think of a thirty-day time improvement, the employee is giving back thirty days of productivity improvement," she says. "So the employee feels better thirty days earlier. Let's assume a productivity improvement by that employee of 20 percent—which is conservative. Take the revenue per employee per year and multiply that by the number of employees affected a year by back pain, and you get the revenue increase that you just benefited from by getting them effective care earlier and helping them move through. That is many millions of dollars for many employers. There's really something here that could shift the paradigm."

As of March 16, 2011, eleven months after the uncomplicated low back pain treatment process had officially commenced, the results of the five metrics were as follows:

- Use of evidence-based medicine 96 percent.
- Patient satisfaction 98 percent.
- Same-day access 98 percent.
- Rapid return to function 100 percent.
- An apparent savings of 10 to 30 percent for patients participating in the value stream process over patients who did not. The cost metric results were preliminary—based on six months of claims—but encouraging. (Most employers of course are thrilled to see a decrease in the rising trend of health care costs. The program's results showed a *negative* trend.)

The Intel team learned a great deal from this program. For one thing it found that same-day access was challenging. There were days when that metric fell to 80 percent, but overall the providers managed to make good on that promise nearly all the time. The team also learned that getting real-time data was very difficult in many instances.

As of late 2011, the Intel-driven marketplace collaborative efforts in Portland had established standardized care for uncomplicated back pain, breast nodules, migraine headaches, and problems with shoulders, knees, and hips. In each case the Virginia Mason model was used as a template. In the case of care for headaches and breast nodules, Virginia Mason's design did not use physicians as initial care providers. In the case of care for shoulders, knees, and hips, Virginia Mason had retained a combined physician and physical therapist visit, and again the Portland collaborative, with the input of Dr. Tom Lorish, delegated initial care to a PT without a physician being present, reducing scheduling and provider cost beyond that which Virginia Mason had achieved.

In addition, Bob Mecklenburg and his Virginia Mason colleagues were on track to create an additional six value streams for the Intel collaborative in 2011. They addressed

- Upper respiratory symptoms
- Screening and prevention
- Depression
- Diabetes
- Abdominal pain
- Chest pain

Thus by the end of 2011, the Intel collaborative was on track to press ahead with improved quality and reduced cost on ten of the most common and expensive conditions for Intel employees.

Although screening and prevention is obviously not a malady, it is nonetheless a high-cost item for Intel and other employers, and Virginia Mason was finding wide variation in how screenings and preventive care were provided; variation that did no good for patients yet was extremely expensive for employers. Upper respiratory issues were found in claims data and hospital records to account for a significant percentage of care patients received, again at a high cost. Mecklenburg's colleague Kim Pittenger had found that Virginia Mason was "spending a great deal of unnecessary physician resources on" screening and prevention and upper respiratory issues. "Both are important," says Mecklenburg, "and patients with upper respiratory problems do need care, but that does not mean they need a physician office visit. With screening and prevention, far too many people are getting unnecessary testing while others are not receiving the care they need. In many cases . . . [appropriate care] does not require a physician visit for screening and prevention—certainly not in many younger, healthy patients with no symptoms, or worries or family history."

## Moving Forward

Pat McDonald started her current journey at Virginia Mason, gaining some initial learning about lean tools that enabled her to manage her plant more efficiently. She then brought the Virginia Mason marketplace collaborative approach to Portland and did so with considerable success. But something else happened in the process of this work. Pat McDonald and her Intel colleagues saw how dysfunctional the American health care system is, and they vowed to play a role in helping to fix it. They now declare that they are on a mission to "transform health care in the United States." And they believe marketplaces collaboratives are a powerful way to help accomplish that goal. Intel is replicating more than the marketplace collaborative model; it is adopting Virginia Mason's vision to transform health care.

Thus the next phase in the work is focusing on expanding the marketplace collaborative concept beyond Intel and Oregon to other major companies in several other states. The goal is to enlist a number of other companies willing to use their purchasing power, along with additional provider groups, who, as Mecklenburg puts it, "don't want to be left out in the cold."

"You pick a topic, define the value stream and your membership, and kick it off," McDonald says. "You observe the work, map it, look at variation and redundancy, eliminate waste, determine a new operating standard, and develop a set of indicators that tell you that you are getting results or not. Then you continuously improve the value stream." Intel's work in Portland has accomplished all that Gary Kaplan had envisioned and that Bob Mecklenburg hoped it would and more. "At this point Intel is clearly demonstrating that an employer-led collaborative implementing value streams is successful," he says. "Providers in other markets with other cultures can replicate the results that the Virginia Mason collaborative achieved. The results in Portland are nearly identical to Seattle. They copied the recipe."

Mecklenburg expects that by spring 2012 the Intel collaborative will have "implemented effective value streams for the top ten most costly conditions, and this will demonstrate in scale the results we have had with the initial value streams. It will show that we can take a huge bite out of the top ten conditions and realize a 20 to 30 percent reduction in costs. *Not a lower trend rate. A reduction in health care costs.* And we will do so by improving quality and speed of access to care."

Virginia Mason's marketplace collaborative work demonstrates progress toward using metrics to manage health care suppliers' performance in achieving standards for quality improvement and cost reduction. It is a supplier management model that can be replicated across Intel and other companies.

## Keys to Doing This Work

- **Know your customer.** Understand the top employers you serve, their workforce demographics, and the health challenges they face in the type of work they do.
- **Know your customer's needs.** Know the top diagnoses of the major employers you serve, including the top issues for your own staff.
- **Establish a clear and measurable definition of quality to guide production, payment, and purchasing of health care.** Work with an employer to define the market-relevant quality they need for the top five diagnoses.
- **Willingness to move ahead.** Be willing to take a leap of faith as a leader and apply the concepts of collaborating, value stream mapping, and putting the patient first to your most complex problems.
- **Engagement of the finance team.** Use the data from finance and purchasing to track and trend progress.

# 3

# CareOregon and Affiliated Clinics

## Producing Health, Changing Lives

Managing health and costs for a Medicaid population is one of the most daunting challenges in health care. We focus in this chapter on CareOregon, a Medicaid managed care plan in Portland, Oregon, which has succeeded in improving the quality of care for its patients while simultaneously controlling costs. Of the 150,000 people for whom CareOregon provides care, 95 percent are at or below the poverty level, nearly half are nonwhite, and about two-thirds are under the age of eighteen.

CareOregon has succeeded not because it has market power—it has very little. It has succeeded by identifying innovative ways to partner with provider organizations and improve the health of its population while reducing use of some of the most expensive forms of care. In its pursuit of the Triple Aim, CareOregon has shifted from serving as a traditional benefit management company to becoming an integrator—a central role through which it collaborates with various providers to improve individual and population health while reducing cost.

"We knew we couldn't do it alone," says Dave Ford, CareOregon's CEO. "We had to pay more and more attention to partnerships in the community for medical services, social services, and more. We've moved from a model . . . [in which we were] just an economic intermediary whose job is to collect money from whoever is purchasing and pay it to providers to [being] an organization that focuses on improvement—on the Triple Aim."

## Crisis 2003

The renaissance at CareOregon began, as is so often the case in health care, with a crisis. In 2003, this health plan that serves a "safety-net population" in Greater Portland stood on the brink of financial collapse. Total cash on hand was sufficient to cover four days of operation. And it was clear that rates for the Medicaid and Medicare populations CareOregon served were not going to get any better and would almost certainly get worse. "We assumed public rates would never keep up with medical inflation and that rate compression would continue over time," says CEO Ford, "which meant that to provide service we had to be a leading-edge innovator on a continuing basis on multiple fronts. The question was could we outperform the rates?" Or, as Ford often says, could they innovate quickly and effectively enough to be able to "outrun the bear?"

Within CareOregon, conversations including Ford, Dr. David Labby, CareOregon's medical director, and others led the organization from focusing on the balance sheet to focusing on the quality of care its patients received. "We were discussing our vision and our mission statement and one of the phrases in it was that we had to have quality care," recalls Ford. "And one of the physicians on our board of directors zeroed in on that and said, 'we don't want quality care. We have to deliver *high-quality* care.'"

And that nuance—that single concept—set CareOregon on a journey to provide nothing less than world-class care to its patients, thus forcing Ford, Labby, and their team to reexamine their work processes, systems—everything.

The challenge was immense. Many if not most of Care-Oregon's patients were poor, unemployed, homeless or in substandard housing, and experiencing depression or mental illness. A significant percentage were addicted to drugs or alcohol. Nearly two-thirds of the adults were afflicted with a chronic illness, and nearly one-third struggled with multiple chronic diseases. As one report put it, the patient population included such cases as "pregnant mothers on methadone; homeless individuals with severe mental illness or substance abuse; patients who are dual-eligible for Medicare and Medicaid and have complex social risk factors; patients with congestive heart failure and other chronic conditions; patients transitioning from hospitals to skilled nursing facilities or home; and patients who have been admitted to the hospital for a psychiatric illness" (Klein & McCarthy, 2010).

In the course of their search for improvement methods, the CareOregon team members have actively sought to learn from other innovators. They have engaged with Göran Henriks and his team from Jönköping County, Sweden; Helen Bevan and her associates in England; the Southcentral Foundation in Alaska; HealthPartners in Minnesota; Group Health in Seattle; and a number of others. They engaged with the Institute for Healthcare Improvement (IHI) and particularly with IHI Senior Fellow Thomas Nolan. At least a year before the 2003 crisis, Ford and his team had begun to center their work around the six elements of quality (safe, effective, patient centered, timely, efficient, and equitable) identified in the Institute of Medicine's 2001 report, *Crossing the Quality Chasm: A New Healthcare System for the 21st Century.* "The *Chasm* report was the basis by which we framed thinking about how, as a payer, to cross over from just being transaction processor to essentially shaping and causing structural change in care delivery systems," says Ford. "*Chasm* said we could no longer accept waste, inefficiency, and lack of patient centeredness."

## CareSupport

David Labby, alluding to Ford's concern with outrunning the bear, says that because payment rates "from the state will never increase as fast as medical costs," CareOregon had to "get at the cost issue by changing the health care delivery system—or we would have a long-term sustainability crisis."

Part of the challenge was that CareOregon was spending 60 percent of its dollars on 12 percent of patients. As a health plan, it could identify those individuals who were in the very high spending category, but what could it do to help those patients improve their health and thereby drive down costs? The most expensive patients, says Labby, were those with multiple chronic conditions "and nobody was coordinating their care. They went to multiple doctors and were left on their own to negotiate their way through the system. Our population didn't often have the skill set to negotiate through the system efficiently on their own behalf. Their care was breaking down and very expensive because they had no support system once they went into treatment. They didn't get support at home or they didn't have stable living conditions and would go back into a facility and languish."

Toward the end of 2003, Ford, Labby, and their team identified this target population and had nurses dig into the patients' cases: Was there family support for a patient? Was he or she ready to change some health behaviors? What were the patient's housing conditions? Did he or she have a consistent and effective relationship with a primary care provider? "We didn't have people with just diabetes or asthma," says Labby. Patients had multiple conditions and required a whole set of services—medical, social, and behavioral.

In 2004, CareOregon created a program called CareSupport, as a way to address the six aims for improvement outlined in *Crossing the Quality Chasm*. The CareSupport program provided case management for these socially and medically complex patients, using plan-based teams of nurses, social workers, and care coordinators assigned to specific primary care practices. Essentially the idea was to identify and work with the patients who were using the most costly care and to improve their outcomes as a means of controlling costs. CareOregon employed predictive modeling in identifying the 3 to 5 percent of its patients at greatest risk, and worked with clinical care teams to focus intensively on helping those patients make improvements.

One method used to propel this population, where too often a sense of hope and motivation is absent, is motivational interviewing. Rebecca Ramsay, CareOregon senior manager of CareSupport & Clinical Programs, introduced motivational interviewing to the CareSupport program. She found that when she began working with clinical teams to identify opportunities to improve outcomes, the case managers would say to her, "this patient just isn't motivated to make any behavior 'changes,' or, there is nothing we can do because this patient won't listen to the advice I am giving him or her." Case managers, already overwhelmed with work, would then close the case. "It bothered me because I heard it so often and knew that we were not going to make a population impact if we didn't find a way to work with these ambivalent patients," says Ramsay. She discussed the issue with a professor she had had in graduate school, and subsequently retained the professor as a consultant for two years "with the goal of building motivational interviewing as a core competency within our case management staff."

The CareOregon team focused on integrating services that required a high degree of coordination, not only among caregivers but also with an array of social service agencies. And team members knew the approach would have to work toward empowering patients to care for themselves to the greatest extent possible. During the two years or so after the crisis—from 2003 to about 2005—they made notable progress as CareOregon's financial situation stabilized, then gradually improved.

As it recovered and revenues picked up, CareOregon went to its network of providers and said the organization was able to pay a bit more money. It would amount to only about $2 per member per month more and CareOregon would still pay at a rate significantly below commercial plans, but it was something. According to Labby the providers' response was, basically, "You pay miserably. Miserable plus $2 is still miserable."

However, the idea was raised that if CareOregon could pay the additional funds to provider organizations as a lump sum grant to be used for innovation, then that money could be significant. Provider budgets were so tight in many cases that they had a difficult time identifying funds with which to experiment. So in 2005, CareOregon created a program called CareSupport System Innovation to fund improvement projects in network provider organizations. Each year, provider organizations would submit program proposals and receive funding. The CareOregon board of directors approved $3 million per year for the initiative, which quickly evolved into a key strategy for helping network providers to transform care.

## The Problem of Producing Health

This much progress was impressive but it got CareOregon only so far. The challenge was that as a health plan CareOregon had only so much leverage to affect the way in which care was delivered to its members. Yet it was clear that the clinical delivery system needed to be more patient-centered than it was. "We had to cross over from what, historically, insurance companies do," says Ford. "We needed to redefine how you produce medicine. We realized we had to collectively change how providers interacted with patients." This notion that a small health plan harbored an ambition to *redefine how you produce medicine* seemed either the height of arrogance or desperation. But it was neither. It was a recognition of reality. CareOregon's cost problems would be solved only if its population's health improved in a measurable way, and that was clearly unlikely under the current system of care.

A central question the leaders at CareOregon wanted to answer was what could they contribute that would have real value to their population. "If it's just paying claims," says Ford, "well, a lot of people can pay claims and ultimately the social value of that is fairly marginal. The question for us is how can we participate in producing health? That is the question we ask. That is the space we need to be in. We were filling in blanks that related to care not given to chronically ill [patients] by creating telephone case managers here at [the] health plan—doing the work and coordination that the clinical practices were not doing. We could see we were dealing with a dysfunctional, uncoordinated primary care system." (In saying this, the CareOregon team was not faulting the clinics, where they knew people were extremely hard working and compassionate, yet they also knew that the clinics were being propelled along a production-based treadmill by a payment system that gave them few alternatives to this production-line approach).

If CareOregon was to survive to be able to care for its population, that had to change. Thus in early 2006, Ford went in search of a sort of Holy Grail—a tried-and-true approach they could replicate at CareOregon. He talked about it with various people he knew from around the country who had been engaged in the quality improvement movement for some time and the name of Southcentral kept coming up. The Southcentral Foundation (SCF) in Anchorage, Alaska, was a health care provider formed and owned by Alaska Natives that provided primary and specialty care in connection with a hospital system for the native Alaska population. The word was getting around that Southcentral, which cared for a population quite similar to CareOregon's, was doing dynamic work. Word was that the foundation was improving the health of its population to the point where it was reducing costs in the highest cost areas—use of the emergency department (ED), specialty care, and hospital admissions—while at the same time improving quality.

## Teaching How to Change Lives

Dave Ford had encountered Dr. Douglas Eby, vice president of medical services at Southcentral Foundation, at various IHI events in the past, and it was clear after some discussions that Eby and his colleagues up in Alaska might well be onto something that could benefit CareOregon. As a result, Ford invited Eby to Portland to speak to the CareOregon board of directors in spring 2006. It proved a pivotal meeting. Eby articulated challenges, frustrations, and hopes that matched those of the CareOregon leaders. But Eby also went much further for he had helped to lead a transformational effort at Southcentral Foundation that had solved some of the most difficult problems that CareOregon was also facing.

That summer, soon after Eby had spoken to the CareOregon board, Ford said to CareOregon medical director David Labby: "We need to go check this out. We're going to take thirty people to Southcentral and you're in charge." Labby quickly set up a scouting mission, traveling to Anchorage during the first week of August 2006 to see the work at Southcentral. He spent several days there with Eby and Michelle Tierney, director of organizational development at Southcentral, learning a good deal about the organization's work. Returning to Portland, he began working to pull the group trip together, with a mounting sense of excitement for what he had seen in Anchorage had "really knocked my socks off."

On August 8, he wrote a memo to the people he hoped would join him on the group trip to Southcentral Foundation, saying that he had come away from his first trip to Southcentral "extremely impressed by the passion about what they do and the professionalism by which they do it." He said that Southcentral's transformation was born of a belief, articulated by Eby, that their core product, facilitated by direct human to human intervention, was "teaching how to changes lives." Labby also noted that Southcentral had successfully (though somewhat painfully) adopted same-day access and created clinical teams to deliver care. Registered nurses had been shifted from clinical silos, where they focused on such things as immunizations, diabetes, and so forth, to working more generally in a team with a physician, a certified medical assistant (CMA), a social worker or behaviorist, and an administrative assistant.

Southcentral Foundation had a total of thirty of these clinical teams working at its center. "The RN case manager works telephonically, supporting both the clinic panel and the village," Labby reported. He wrote that the focus at Southcentral was

> on preventive and chronic disease care; there are electronic tools/ profiles that allow the team to know their sub populations of diabetics, asthmatics etc so that guideline based care and preventive care can be reliably delivered. RN expected to ensure that those in the chronic disease registries get all guideline recommended care and that preventive services are offered. The MD/RN/CMA team review schedules before and during clinic sessions to make sure they are prepared to offer all recommended services during the appointment so no opportunity is missed to deliver needed care. The RN case manager also has disease registries that inform her of patients who need to be brought in for gaps in recommended care. The result has been impressive documented improvements in chronic disease management in diabetes, asthma, and even chronic pain as well as improvements in delivery of general health preventive services such as mammography and colon cancer screening . . .

Labby's memo provided background for those planning to join the trip to Anchorage, scheduled for August 29 to September 1. The goal of the trip was to try, as Labby wrote, to assess "the applicability of the SCF model, or parts of that model, to CareOregon and its network." The delegation heading north included a CareOregon team as well as representatives from four clinics in the Portland area that provided the bulk of the care for CareOregon members—Legacy Clinic Emanuel, the Multnomah County Health Department, the Richmond Clinic at Oregon Health & Science University, and the Virginia Garcia Memorial Health Center.

A couple of Oregon state legislators went along as well. The four clinics sent teams that included both clinicians (some of them medical directors) and administrators. Many members of the delegation had had an opportunity to hear Eby talk about Southcentral's work during one of his visits to Portland and word of this new approach had spread rapidly. Thus everyone on the trip had at least a basic sense of what was happening at SCF.

The delegation's visit began with a presentation by Doug Eby and other staff members, including those responsible for training as well as behavioral health. The delegation toured the facility and saw the clinical teams in action, taking particular note of primary care team members—physician, nurse, medical assistant, and social worker or behaviorist—positioned together in the workplace enabling them to engage with one another and function as a cohesive unit throughout the day. The delegation saw care managers who dealt directly with their patients—who knew their patients' histories and challenges in detail. They witnessed situations where a care manager, receiving a phone call from a patient, would consult with the doctor or nurse or social worker seated a few feet away and then guide the patient. At one point the CareOregon team members witnessed a physician who was returning to the area where he worked with other colleagues, pointing to the care manager and remarking, "She doesn't work for me. I really work for her!"

The delegation also met with some Southcentral Foundation *customer owners*, Alaska Native people who had experienced care under both the old and new systems. Ford, Labby and their fellow visitors found it extremely moving to hear stories indicating how deeply proud the people were in the excellence of the Indian Health Service as embodied in Southcentral Foundation. Ford says: "It was so clear that they had this tremendous pride in this organization—that the Southcentral system had a special place in their community."

## Recognizing a Better Way to Practice Medicine

The trip was proof of the belief that Ford and Labby had expressed prior to traveling to Anchorage—that hearing about the Southcentral work was one thing but that seeing it firsthand on the shop floor was vastly more meaningful. "People were on fire about the possibilities," says Ford.

As they had seen at Southcentral, world-class care was about teamwork, standards, reaching out to patients, and as Eby had said, "teaching how to change lives." Everything they saw reinforced what they had heard from Eby over and over: that the core of their new system had to be about creating "continuous healing relationships" between patients and their provider teams. "Effective medical care is not about pills and procedures," Eby would repeat, "but about building relationships, walking with someone else in their journey over time."

After he had returned from Anchorage, David Labby put some of his thoughts on paper:

> What we saw was not health care as we know it. Open Access: patients who could see their assigned doctor the same day as long as they called by 4:30 PM. Team Care: doctors who work side by side with case management nurses to do whatever is needed to help their patients. This might be an office visit if you really NEED to see the doctor; but it could be a telephone call back if you just have a question. If you do come [in] it is probably to see a doctor you have known for a long time and who knows you and your family. Each team is assigned a panel of about 1000 patients and patients are encouraged to sign up as families so . . . [teams] get to know patients better. . . .
>
> During visits, there is plenty of time to go over all your concerns, as well as do whatever health screening is due so you don't have to come back. Doctors aren't paid per visit, so there is no incentive to have you come in if you don't need [to] or to come back if everything can be done when you are there. Behavioral health

providers are on site to address whatever mental health issues might arise during the visit, so no one in distress need wait to get help.

If you don't come in you might also get a call that your health screening, or a checkup for some chronic condition, is due since they track all their patients' health needs on a data base and reach out to help patients stay healthy. And it works: decreasing rates of hospitalizations and ED visits, near world-class immunization and preventive measure rates, and excellent outcomes for people with chronic conditions such as diabetes and asthma.

Although the delegation was deeply impressed, there was also concern. It was so different from the way things worked in Portland that one of the CareOregon board members said that it would be great to do, "but I can't see how we can get from where we are today to *this*."

But they had to try. Labby says that before their plane took off from Anchorage the delegation members had moved from asking, "Should we do this?" to asking, "How could we not do this?"

The board member, however, had raised a very good question: How *could* CareOregon get from here to there? And the only possible answer was that it would have to be done through collaboration with the providers who had accompanied the CareOregon team to Anchorage. CareOregon had no control over what happened in any of the clinics serving its patients. Thus any transformation in care delivery would have to come about as the result of enthusiasm on the part of the provider organizations. And it was not as simple as collaborating with one provider group. Five clinics would have to take on the challenge—five clinics that had never before all worked together.

But there was a powerful sense of possibility among the returning clinicians and administrators from the provider organizations. They had seen a new way of delivering care, and they wanted it for their patients. Clinicians talked about the team-based care, including the behavioral health component connected to primary care. They talked about continuous healing relationships with patients. "Doctors saw the way things worked at Southcentral," says Labby, "and said, 'Of course! This is the way I want to be able to practice. This is why I went into medicine.'"

At the end of the three-day site visit to Anchorage, the group had committed to finding a way to test whether Southcentral's model could be re-created in multiple clinics attached to various organizations, each with different resources and somewhat different patient populations.

There were several immediate issues. CareOregon had a significantly different relationship with its contracted network than the Southcentral leadership had with its staff; and although one could visit and see what Southcentral had put in place, there was no blueprint or set of guidelines for re-creating Southcentral's model. Nonetheless, it was clear to the delegation that there were five key components to the system they had seen over the past few days: (1) team-based care, (2) proactive panel management, (3) patient-centered care, (4) advanced access, and (5) behavioral health integration. To build the kind of robust medical home they had just seen, clinics would have to be willing to commit to implementing all of these components.

## A Collaborative Effort

As the work began in earnest in Portland, the teams involved were mindful of the advice Doug Eby and his team had conveyed regarding the general approach—that tackling the work piecemeal was not likely to succeed. "They made it clear that you cannot do this as single projects," says Ford. "You had to do . . . [all the parts] at once. And the reason they gave was that if you do them in a linear way instead of concurrently, . . . there are so many different pieces that get involved that you will run out of commitment and time to get it done and you would fail." The team at Southcentral had tried to work on improvement projects in a sequential fashion and had too often found that once the team completed work on one project and moved on to the next, the completed work was not sustained. For CareOregon to change the way its patients received care meant undertaking whole system change all at once—something vastly more complex than the leadership team had ever before attempted. "We had had some important projects in the past with some success," says Labby. "A program for diabetes, for example, but it didn't change the fundamentals and we needed to be more aspirational." Ford,

Labby, and others believed that they needed a new model of care that would give them the quality and cost results they needed to achieve.

Among the most important lessons the CareOregon team learned from Southcentral was that, as Ford put it, "there was a process by which teams could treat populations together in a much more supportive way than . . . a single doctor in an encounter-based practice [could]." This was the heart of the matter—the need to create teams and establish best practices and standard work for them to implement.

CareOregon and the clinics that treated its patients formed a collaborative with the purpose of adapting the Southcentral approach to their work in Portland. Clinics interested in being pilot sites for the new work—and all the clinics represented on the Anchorage trip as well as a fifth clinic, Central City Concern, were interested—submitted proposals to CareOregon in mid-November 2006. CareOregon had set aside funding to get the program off the ground, which meant paying each clinic enough to set up internal pilot teams to try to adapt the Southcentral approach. The payments from CareOregon to fund the pilot teams were critically important.

"You need to create capacity in order to change," says Dr. David Shute, of GreenField Health in Portland. Shute had had experience in setting up and guiding learning collaboratives, and he was hired by Labby to help structure the multiorganizational collaborative along the lines described in the IHI white paper *The Breakthrough Series: IHI's Collaborative Model for Achieving Breakthrough Improvement* (Institute for Healthcare Improvement, 2003). "If you are running full speed trying to see patients and do the basics, you have no excess capacity," Shute continues. "One of the first steps was to create new capacity, and that is part of what the funding did—create capacity to begin testing the changes." In addition to the financial support, CareOregon provided a central coordinating function, project management staff, technical support, and improvement training for clinics working on applying the new model.

The clinics joining in the collaboration differed in a variety of ways. The Cornelius branch of the Virginia Garcia Memorial Health Center, for example, had a high percentage of migrant farmworkers among its patients, and Central City Concern had a clinic for the homeless that had roots as a drug and alcohol treatment facility and offered robust behavioral health and other services. The Richmond Clinic at Oregon Health & Science University served a multiethnic urban population and had a family medicine residency, and Legacy Clinic Emanuel served a major African American community and included an internal medicine residency program through which many young physicians passed during their time as residents.

Although the CareOregon team had a fairly deep understanding of the Southcentral work, they needed to dig deeper in order to create a curriculum to teach workers in all the participating clinical pilot sites. David Labby and Rebecca Ramsay returned to Southcentral in September 2006 with the goal of engaging in close observation for the purpose of designing a curriculum, a teaching blueprint, for the Portland clinical teams. Labby and Ramsay shadowed Southcentral care teams and interviewed leaders and staff to look more deeply into the ways Southcentral's model functioned on the ground. Using what they learned, Labby and Ramsay put together an initial change package that they would apply back in Portland, including specific role training for case managers, behavioral health providers, nurses, and doctors.

## Primary Care Renewal

Meanwhile Ford and his team had put together a proposal for a program they called Primary Care Renewal. Essentially, the idea was to create a patient-centered medical home for all their members. Ford described it as shifting primary care so it was no longer the responsibility of a physician working relatively independently and instead became the responsibility of a coordinated delivery team that would know and serve all of a patient's health needs, with each need being addressed in the lowest cost setting that the team deemed appropriate.

Why call this program Primary Care Renewal? The answer, Labby wrote at the time, was that "this is the way those who went in to health care thought they would be practicing when they started training. It is called 'renewal' because it is based on reestablishing the personal relationship most of us want from the health care system. It is called 'renewal' because it might be one small Oregon step in moving the most expensive heath care system in the world toward the most satisfying and effective system the world can offer."

Funding from the CareOregon improvement program was essential. CareOregon was, after all, asking clinics to do more work and to do things not typically paid for in the fee-for-service reimbursement model. The team knew that the work would require additional staff—behavioral health specialists if nothing else. And because CareOregon was proposing to build a patient-centered medical home where the full array of patients' needs could be met and where the caregivers got to know the patients in their panel very well, all the people on each clinical care team would be "practicing at the top of their license or capability," says Ramsay. Ramsay says CareOregon pushed hard to make sure that all the work that could be performed effectively by nurses, medical assistants, social workers, pharmacists, and others was, in fact, performed by those personnel. This would leave the physicians more time to focus on the kinds of issues for which doctors are trained. The result, at least in theory, would be more time for each patient with some member of the primary care team and more *impactful* time with his or her doctor. "We were saying to the clinics that we want to transform primary care in our community and based on what we saw at SCF, here are the five principles that we believe should guide that transformation," says Ramsay.

The collaborative was to be launched with a *charter meeting* to agree on direction and goals and decide on an initial set of common measures. The collaborative learning process would include consultation and guidance from experienced faculty (who would be retained by CareOregon as consultants), and training and instruction for engaging in panel and case management work, providing open access, and integrating behavioral health into care. CareOregon would provide, in effect, a moveable learning and development center. Finally, the pilot teams would convene every six weeks at a formal *learning session* to report on common measures and discuss progress.

By the first week in February 2007, the pilot teams were chosen, the guidelines and structure going forward were defined, and the collaborative was ready to launch. At the charter meeting on February 6, Labby, echoing a guiding principle from Dr. Paul Batalden of Dartmouth Medical School, a founding board member of IHI, emphasized to the assembled pilot teams that going forward everyone would have two jobs: "Job 1 is to provide care," he said. "Job 2 is to improve care." The goal, he explained, was to accelerate progress by sharing experience on an ongoing basis and to spread Primary Care Renewal beyond the pilot sites.

All members of the clinic pilot teams went through a training process under the tutelage of consultant Jane Norman. Norman had many years of experience in quality improvement and management, which she drew on to teach the clinic teams how to carry out the planned improvements in their care delivery systems.

In March 2007, staff from CareOregon and teams from the participating Primary Care Renewal clinics convened for a discussion. Altogether, there were ninety people in the room, and the teams represented had never before worked with each other. Ford and Labby spoke to the assembled group and explained that in a fundamental sense Primary Care Renewal was a patient-centered medical home pilot collaborative between CareOregon and the assembled provider groups. The hope and belief was that Primary Care Renewal would provide more effective care for patients, reenergize providers, and make primary care more attractive to graduating medical students as a way to make a significant difference in patient's lives. They also stated explicitly their hope that more effective primary care would decrease unnecessary, high-cost utilization, such as ED visits or hospitalizations, allowing both more investment in primary care infrastructure and a more sustainable health care system generally.

The team-based approach they were using was the program's foundation. Ford says the collaborative moved over time from *yestercare*, which he defined as "heroic/expert, professional-centric, rescue/late stage, population indifferent" care toward *futurecare*, which he defined as Triple Aim balanced, whole system metrics, population accountable, team based, and postheroic.

"I think it is a fairly profound notion that CareOregon was moving from the traditional health plan role to trying to catalyze change in the provider community," says David Shute. "This was new territory for health plans. They were making robust changes not only in how clinics deliver care but actually redefining what the product is."

Traditionally, the clinic product was treating sickness in a visit-based setting and CareOregon was asking the clinics to get better at that. But they were also asking the clinics to do more—for example to become proactive about wellness and to integrate behavioral health into primary care. And the clinics were eager to do so. "It was really getting at what people wanted to do," says Labby. "That's what created the infectious element of spread."

The new Primary Care Renewal approach comprised the following five foundational components that the delegation had identified at Southcentral Foundation.

### Team-Based Care

Dr. Beth Averbeck, associate medical director for primary care at HealthPartners in Minnesota, put it succinctly: "Primary care is a team sport." Primary Care Renewal was shifting visit-based care to a care model offering more prevention, wellness, and outreach and requiring care managers, panel managers, and behavioral health specialists as well as doctors and nurses.

Learning and adapting to new roles was not a simple matter. Going from being reactive—waiting for patients to make appointments and come into the clinic—to being proactive—managing the health of the population and reaching out to patients in need of services—was a huge challenge. But the logic of the new approach was clear. Many duties previously handled by a doctor could clearly be accomplished by other team members—filling prescriptions, updating tests and screenings, and much more.

"Most, if not all, of the safety-net primary care clinics had acknowledged that their nurses were being underutilized and many were not happy with the largely technical and administrative tasks they were doing on a daily basis," says Ramsay. "Team-based care offered the nurses an opportunity to step into the professional role they were prepared and excited to take on." This, ideally, would leave the physician to do what he or she had been trained to do: complex medical decision making.

### Proactive Panel Management

The idea of proactive panel management harkens back to old-fashioned doctor-patient relationships in a way. Doctors had to know the patients for whom they were responsible, and patients had to know who their doctors were. But proactive management of a panel of patients means all the care team members have to know their patients and vice versa. For the CareOregon collaborative this required not only a new approach and culture but also data systems that enabled fast-moving population management.

"The data piece is huge," says Labby. "With data you can act on the Triple Aim." Establishing proactive panel management involved creating a tool listing all panel members and essential information about the services they required and standardizing the visit so that a patient's screening needs were anticipated and set up beforehand, allowing the actual visit time to be used more productively. This approach required panel managers to scan their lists each day to anticipate their patients' needs. It also required panel managers to reach out between visits to their patients to engage them in education and in getting updated services, and it meant setting manageable panel sizes. For an urban population with homeless patients, for example, this meant a panel size of about 900 to 1,200 patients. Internal medicine panels ranged from 1,200 to 1,500 patients. "Panel management became a new role for [medical assistants and licensed practical nurses]," says Ramsay. "We even discovered from other health systems that college students can do a fabulous job at panel management."

This frontline work was very much Triple Aim focused, says Ramsay, involving "mapping the needs of a population within the context of a particular health care setting and discovering the most efficient and effective way of meeting those needs."

### Patient-Centered Care

At the Southcentral Foundation leaders had sought to listen to the voice of the patient in many different ways—surveys, focus groups, discussions with people in waiting rooms, and more. They had even engaged the patients in the design of the physical plant and employed symbols of health and caring in building an efficient, functional, and beautiful facility for the community. "A rich feedback system is essential," says David Labby. The CareOregon collaborative sought to install similar patient feedback loops. When the CareOregon team members looked at patient satisfaction surveys, they found that most did not get at the key elements they were trying to build into the model. This led to the creation of new tools to assess the program's patient centeredness and of new ways to evaluate the patient's experience of care.

### Advanced Access

On one level advanced access meant that the clinics would work to keep about 30 percent of their slots open each day for immediate appointments. But the collaborative also wanted to reach beyond this traditional definition and to think in terms of creating more access in a variety of ways, including telephone calls, e-mails, group visits, and more. If building relationships was to be the core of the system, the clinics would need multiple ways for people to connect, methods driven by what works for the patients and not just for the providers. Labby defines advanced access as IHI has defined it in the past, from the patient's point of view: *all the care I want and need when and how and where I need it.* Says Labby, "It's the backbone of the relationship."

### Behavioral Health Integration

Integrating behavioral health into primary care was a huge challenge, but given the nature of the problems faced by the population CareOregon serves, it was essential. However, the behavioral health piece of the Primary Care Renewal program proved difficult to crack initially. Because a primary care role for a behavioral health specialist did not exist in the clinics, the collaborative was starting almost from scratch.

"When people were hired into that role, they figured it out for themselves," says Labby. "Their role in the clinics had to be very solution and action based, and it was hard for some of the specialists to give up their role as therapists." In fact some people hired as behavioral health specialists did not last very long in the new role because of their experience as therapists. The behavioral health specialists embedded in primary care teams were not asked to be psychoanalysts so much as coaches for problem solving. They would focus on brief behavioral interventions—straightforward, cognitive behavioral therapy. For therapists accustomed to deep dives with each patient, the new role could seem fleeting and unsatisfying. Those unable to give up the traditional therapy model eventually moved on.

But almost from the start, most of the men and women hired as behavioral health specialists in the clinics began meeting and exchanging ideas and information. They formed a supportive learning community that was sustained over time. One of the keys to success was that these behavioral health providers became quite effective at showing how helpful they could be to primary care physicians. Ramsay says that from the start these specialists were skillful about what amounted to marketing their services to primary care physicians—helping doctors to understand how behavioral health providers could play an important value-added role in patient treatment.

## Clinic Pilot Teams

*The Breakthrough Series: IHI's Collaborative Model for Achieving Breakthrough Improvement* defines a collaborative as a "short-term (6- to 15-month) learning system that brings together a large number of teams from hospitals or clinics to seek improvement in a focused topic area" (Institute for Healthcare Improvement, 2003). They rely on adaptation of existing knowledge locally with subsequent spread to multiple settings to accomplish a common aim. Collaboratives are action- and results-oriented structures where "all teach and all learn." Effective collaboratives create a sense of both familiarity and comfort—as collaborators help and support one another—while at the same time they foster competition among the teams.

CareOregon used the IHI model as a way to organize the five clinics within a learning collaborative. Each of the clinics participating in the collaborative selected a pilot team of four to six people. Typically, the teams comprised a clinician, whose role involved diagnosis and complex care plan oversight as well as leadership and consultation with the team; a nurse case manager to coordinate and provide care; a clerical assistant to support the case manager and provide administrative help to the team; a medical assistant to conduct screenings and move patients in and out of visits; and a behavioral health specialist.

The learning collaborative brought the clinics together to share ideas, and as Shute says, "sharing what you have learned and new ideas keeps the energy up and keeps people moving forward. It also accelerates the rate of learning." Sherril Gelmon, a Portland State University professor who had experience with teaching process improvement to health care professionals, provided the framework for the pilot teams on how to conduct PDSA (plan-do-study-act) improvement cycles. Her work complemented the work of Jane Norman. From the start CareOregon wanted the teams to pursue change in their work around the five guidelines (team-based care, proactive panel management, patient-centered care, advanced access, and behavioral health integration), but it did not dictate how the teams would do that. "These were principles," says Labby, "and we told the pilots, 'You figure out how best to reach these goals.' There was a lot of experimentation and a lot of the pilots' sharing what they learned. Our thought was that these are guiding principles and we have to let people apply them in their setting the way that works best for them." In this the CareOregon team was guided by what Ramsay describes as a "foundational principle of process improvement—that the people doing the work are the best people to figure out how to improve the work."

## The Importance of Training and Instruction

Dave Ford, David Labby, and their colleagues had come away from Southcentral understanding clearly that quality training and instruction was foundational to any improvement work. Southcentral, in fact, had drawn some of its training methods from Jönköping County health system in Sweden, where Göran Henriks runs a well-known improvement and innovation center called Qulturum.

"Southcentral is very committed to workforce development," says Labby. "That was a real *aha* for us—that you can't just do it; that you have to teach people how to do change. Jane Norman came in and taught the basics of improvement. We hired her both to help us as an organization build our internal development center and also to train people to do Primary Care Renewal work in the clinics."

Engaging in the training and instruction with Norman was a requirement for all participating pilot teams. Once the training of the pilot teams was completed, each team designated two individuals to serve as improvement coaches, and they received additional training from Norman. The process improvement coaches on each team would lead PDSA improvement cycles on a variety of aspects of care management. For example, Labby says, a simple PDSA cycle sought to "decrease interruptions of the providers while they are seeing patients. So the team would set up a tracking system to see how many interruptions occurred over a day or several days; then look at what [these interruptions] were for and lump them together into categories; then make a few changes in workflows to handle some of the issues differently, for example, defining what is urgent versus what can wait, who else can answer the question, [and so forth]."

Citing another example, Labby notes that provider teams were learning to review charts before visits, in an effort to identify opportunities to provide needed preventive or chronic care. The question then arose of whether placing "a checklist of services to be reviewed in the chart [would] help? Would more needed services be provided if there was some standard way to record what is due, even if there is an EMR? Many of the teams tried different tools and workflows to do this 'scrubbing' work."

Rebecca Ramsay was integrally involved in the Primary Care Renewal collaborative. She says the training sessions got down to practical basics including teaching pilot teams about "huddling, teamwork, division of labor, understanding what could be delegated, process work, how you scrubbed the chart. So that rather than just taking the onslaught of patients coming in, you would begin the day looking at all patients and make decisions about what people needed. The idea was to move from encounter focus to looking at people longitudinally."

## Fundamental Change

The shift to a new approach was not expected to be easy, and it was not. The difference between treating each patient who comes through the door of the clinic one at a time versus focusing more broadly on population management—and getting to know each patient—was immensely challenging. "This is not a series of PDSA cycles," says Debra Read, Care Innovations senior evaluation associate who was also involved with the Primary Care Renewal work. "It's a real shift to how everything is organized and structured."

Labby thinks of the change as cultural and structural. "The old model was that all clinicians were in a condominium practice where each doctor does his own thing and nobody knows what anybody else is doing," he says. "There is a parallel support system for clinicians—basically condominium staff who take patients and put them in front of the doctor in a room and then take the patients afterward and do what the doctor says and take them away. We're moving from that individualist, heroic practice with a support structure to a system with a comprehensively designed division of labor and integrated workflows, all directed at getting the best health outcomes for the population of people served."

Debra Read says that before Primary Care Renewal most of the practices had no idea how many patients with diabetes they had, for example. But with a population focus, data become the clinic's lifeblood and data reveal precisely which patients are in an appropriate place and which are not.

In CareOregon's new learning center, Rebecca Ramsay started a learning collaborative to teach nurses the principles of population care management. Initially this shift was not easy for nurses at the clinics, who had generally been in a triage role. Through this care management learning collaborative, nurses acquired face-to-face care management techniques that would help them guide patients to the kind of changes that could improve their health. "The problem was the difference between how we at the health plan see things from a population point of view and how clinicians see it in an episodic world," says Ramsay. "Initially it was a struggle to convert nurses and case managers to focus on chronic and complex management."

Coaches met every other week to share results and help coach one another. Norman phoned into these sessions in an effort to guide the coaches and their teams. With this system, every pilot team knew what every other team was working on at any given time and important lessons were shared. The process improvement coaches quickly bonded into a cohesive learning group and became the glue of the collaborative.

In addition to the coaches' sessions every other week, there was a meeting of the full collaborative team every six weeks, hosted by CareOregon and led by Labby. In these sessions, members of each pilot group would discuss what they had been working on and what their major lessons were. Best practices were quickly identified and shared with the full collaborative. Then the members of each pilot team reported to the group what they planned to tackle—and how they would measure it—in the next six weeks.

"This collective learning model was really, really effective," says Labby. "We'd focus on what they had been most successful with that they wanted to share with the other pilot teams and what they were struggling with." There was also much experimentation. Ideas that seemed promising sometimes worked beautifully and other times did not. "People would come in and say at one meeting that a particular approach they were using was the coolest thing ever," says Labby, "and come back six weeks later and say, 'that was the stupidest thing we ever came up with.'"

## From Pilots to Spread

Toward the end of 2007 and beginning of 2008, it was clear something special was happening at the pilot sites. There was a sense of joy and satisfaction among the pilot teams that the clinicians who were not on those teams could not help but notice. "The people who were not on the pilot teams were observing their pilot-team colleagues operating in a more collaborative, team-based approach," says Ramsay. "They were seeing huddling and the teams working together as a unit versus the traditional form of practice where you are doing your own thing." Moreover, physicians on the pilot teams made no secret of their belief that Primary Care Renewal enabled them to do a better job of taking care of patients and elevated their own sense of professional satisfaction.

"Spread sort of broke out," says Labby.

It was clear to CareOregon leaders that if Primary Care Renewal was going to take root and spread in all the clinics, it would be because the organizations involved wanted it and owned the process, not because it was orchestrated for them externally. "The organization leaders from the clinics had to own it," says Labby. "It had to be theirs. It couldn't be ours. They had to be able to run their own collaborative or similar implementation model in their organizations so that this became their new business model."

The formal breakthrough collaborative was ended and replaced by a steering committee made up of two people from each of the organizations participating in the collaborative—usually an operations person and the medical director. The committee members met regularly to report on their progress, to share the methods they were using to spread the Primary Care Renewal model throughout their organizations, and to discuss common challenges. None of the clinics, as it turned out, completely reproduced the *Breakthrough Series* model, but all had their version of it adapted to the needs of their own organization. All of the participants created a method of spreading and sharing learning throughout their organizations.

Labby recalls that there were constant challenges. "Just because you say it's a team model not everybody wants to be on a team," he says. "How do you deal with a team that is not functioning well? What if a team is passive aggressive and not working well? Whose job is it to go in and coach the team? How do you do that and who does it? How do you manage change? How do you spread what you have done in the pilots? One analogy was do you give them quiche, or eggs and the other ingredients?"

There was both art and science to establishing the new system, and it became clear that good teaching and providing the teams with a sense of empowerment was the right mix. The message was essentially that—we will teach you what we have learned that we believe works really well for improved primary care. You have the power to implement this, to adapt it, or to reshape it in a way that works best for you and your team.

In eighteen months, CareOregon's Primary Care Renewal project had spread from five to twenty-six teams. Each team has built on the experiences of others with continuous adaptation. In fact, Ford says, some practices have driven the medical home model further out, to parts of their business beyond Medicaid.

## The Challenge of Behavioral Health Integration

Perhaps the biggest challenge to the providers involved integrating behavioral health into primary care. This meant shifting staff members around and having a reliable process to get patients in need of help into the right hands. Some clinics had staff they could redeploy to work with patients—a social worker, for example—and others hired someone new for the role. But "once the organizations got people on board there was a lot of confusion among behavioralists about what exactly they were supposed to do," says Labby. Then, as we mentioned earlier, in the summer of 2007, the behavioral health consultants pulled themselves together as group and began meeting each month to share stories and problems. They became another learning collaborative, one where the ongoing question was, "How do we learn how to do this better?"

It was essential to make headway with behavioral health, says Labby, because behavioral issues drive much of health outcomes and conditions such as anxiety and depression were "extremely common" in the CareOregon population. But the solution was not as simple as antianxiety or antidepressant medication. "A lot of things are important for recovery from depression," says Labby. "People who are depressed don't do much. They are not active. They retreat into a smaller space and become socially isolated. Instead of meds you can schedule pleasurable activity, ask the patient what they really enjoy. 'OK, what about trying to walk the dog three times a week?' You get it going. 'I'll call you in a week.' You try and get at what's bothering them. People can have mistaken assumptions and get stuck in a thought pattern. 'Is it really true that your life is over and there is nothing possible for you?' It's helping people get unstuck."

Treatment for such patients, says Labby, isn't about "'let's talk about your childhood and how stressful the environment was,' but what can we do now. Sometimes it's a PDSA cycle of therapy." One PDSA cycle resulted in an important bit of progress on getting patients to see the behavioral health specialists. Clinics found that when doctors referred patients for mental health appointments, a majority typically would not show up for the appointment. Patients felt somewhat stigmatized by "mental health" or "behavioral health" characterization and thus shied away from going to the appointment.

The Richmond Clinic found a much more effective method, says David Shute. "It is a warm handoff where a member of the team walks the patient down the hall and says, 'Let me introduce you to Nancy. She is part of our team.' It's tremendously effective because you don't leave it to the patient to remember and take the initiative. The key piece is, by doing a personal introduction, you've established that relationship with the mental health provider."

The inclusion of behavioral health in the mix has "fundamentally changed the way we do primary care," says Labby. "So much of what we deal with is not physical medicine. We know health outcomes are driven by social and behavioral determinants and that what we do on [the] medical side is secondary to that." Labby cites an analysis by Steven Schroeder (2007) suggesting that even if medical care for all people was perfect and everyone in the population received evidence-based treatment, it would decrease early mortality by only 10 percent. However, continuing with Schroeder's statistics, Labby notes that if everybody had perfect social behavior—did not smoke, drink, become obese, or live in substandard housing—it would reduce early mortality by 40 percent. "All of these things are bigger than medical care," says Labby. "The medical system is a fix-it shop. All we do is fix things that are broken. We do not really prevent much of what causes ill health."

The behavioral work has proven so important Labby says, that "if this whole thing fell apart and clinicians could keep one thing it would be the behavioral piece."

## The Multnomah County Experience

With 35,000 patients, the Multnomah County Health Department was the largest participant in the CareOregon collaborative. Susan Kirchoff, director of health centers operations at the Multnomah County Health Department, was attracted to the Primary Care Renewal approach because she believed it had the potential to create the kind of medical home that would enable ongoing relationships between empowered patients and the health care team. She believed that the route to coordinated and integrated care was through provider teams who were accessible and who had, as she put it, "a whole person orientation."

Multnomah's pilot site was Mid County Health Center in southeast Portland—the health department's largest clinic and one where only about a third of the patients were native English speakers. The clinic also included a refugee center.

An initial problem in the county was a lack of patient panels. Patients related to a particular clinic rather than a specific primary care provider. Thus patients did not know who their doctor was and doctors did not know who their patients were. Empaneling patients was an important first step.

The next big step involved what Kirchoff calls the process to "co-locate" the provider teams—that is, put all team members together in one room. Each team consisted of two physicians, two medical assistants, a panel manager, a clerical assistant, and a behavioral health specialist. The purpose of the co-location was to facilitate communication among team members. Part of the challenge in the process of setting the teams up in the same clinic space involved architectural constraints and another part of the challenge was resistance on the part of some providers who wanted to continue having an office in an area with other providers. But fairly quickly and without much difficulty, the teams were settled into a location together, and Kirchoff could see that it was an important step forward. "It felt like a real page-turner," she says. "It seemed like we were really ready to change. We had a history of making changes that weren't sustained but this was different."

The teams in the Multnomah County pilot clinic relied on a rich data set (the clinic had just completed the installation of new electronic health records) to identify patients in need of various prevention and wellness interventions. The teams also created a dashboard with cost, quality, and access measures, and real-time access to the data set helped them measure as their work proceeded. "Proactive outreach to patients with diabetes, hypertension, asthma, and more was a big change for us," says Kirchoff. "Before that we were focused on the individual visit." The new approach meant big changes for provider teams, yet it felt fairly comfortable to them within a matter of a few months. They were more proactive than before in many ways, including reviewing the schedule the day before and reaching out to patients between visits. They redesigned their approach to setting up appointments and scheduling providers to improve access and continuity. A big step came in improving call management so that when patients phoned in they spoke directly with a member of *their* care team. The pilot teams became more proactive about engaging patients and families both with face-to-face discussions about patient expectations and levels of satisfactions. A newly redesigned patient satisfaction survey was also used.

As much as anything, the integration of behavioral health into the primary care clinic made an enormous difference. With the new "warm handoff"—which the Multnomah team adopted from the learning collaborative—the no-show rate was significantly reduced. "The PCPs loved it," Kirchoff says.

At the same time providers were challenged by having to increase the number of patients they saw, due to budget issues, but despite this, within a few months the teams agreed that they were providing better care for their patients—much better in many instances. "About four to six months into the pilot it became clear the new approach was starting to work," says Kirchoff. "We started to see a few clinical results changing and patient satisfaction improving."

In the fall of 2007, all of Multnomah County's primary care doctors gathered for a meeting where the pilot teams presented their assessment of the Primary Care Renewal work to date. The enthusiasm was palpable. Team members spoke of improved clinical results and deepening relationships with and understanding of patients. They talked about the real value of the behavioral health component. They talked about having an identified panel of patients and about the impact of outreach and between-visit care. A patient with multiple medical issues stood in front of the meeting recounting how she had been laid off and had lost her commercial health insurance. Moving to the public health plan, she was fearful about getting good care, but she said that at the Multnomah County clinic, she got better care than she had under her old commercial plan.

Kirchoff and her team began to spread the Primary Care Renewal process from the original pilot site to other Multnomah clinic sites in the fall of 2007. They proceeded carefully, one clinic at a time, starting with "readiness visits" to determine the specific work that would be needed to prepare the clinic for the new method of delivering care. "We spread according to readiness," says Kirchoff. In all, the Multnomah County Health Department spread the method to eight clinics over a two-year period. In each clinic, Kirchoff and other leadership team members were intensively involved for the first ninety days of the transition period and then they gradually backed away as the clinics gained confidence in the new processes and were able to continue to improve with less direct support. "We've learned how to pace change more effectively," Kirchoff says. "You have to give people time and space. If you move too fast you have to go back and redo it, and we had to do that on a couple of occasions. In the early phases we didn't give people enough time to really embed the change in their practice before we launched something new."

Although it was clear that leadership was essential to sustaining the gains, Kirchoff says the hardest part of the spread was shifting to a team concept of care. "It was about the teams really learning how to work together," she says. "You can't underestimate the importance of that, and you have to keep going back and revisiting it as new team members are added."

The Multnomah clinical teams benefited greatly from their inclusion in the CareOregon learning collaborative, and they also engaged in ongoing learning collaboratives internally. For example, they would convene all panel managers from all the clinics to discuss the issues and challenges they faced—and to share ideas and best practices. Behavioral health specialists and nurses were also brought together for this purpose. "When you get forty-five nurses all together in one room and they teach each other, it doesn't take much facilitation," says Kirchoff. "They really enjoy learning from one another."

The next group to be engaged in the collaborative learning approach were the providers, who until recently had met together only for clinical education.

## Tackling Disease Management at the Clinic Level

Disease management was an essential element of the Primary Care Renewal (PCR) approach. It would not only improve care between visits but it was also a required element if CareOregon was to earn National Committee for Quality Assurance (NCQA) accreditation—the gold seal of approval. Traditionally, health plans assigned disease management responsibility to outside vendors. Patients who would benefit from disease management intervention would be identified, and the outside vendor would contact them in the hope that they would engage in the program. But Rebecca Ramsay thought that it made no sense for CareOregon to farm out the disease management function. She had been working diligently with the clinic teams on a variety of training initiatives, and she believed that the clinic teams themselves could be capable, with some additional training, of handling disease management on their own. Moreover, "the idea of vendors was not well-received by the PCR providers," says Ramsay. "The vendor call center may be located anywhere and they are calling your patients and coaching, but they have no connection to the primary care team responsible for that patient. They are completely disconnected from the primary care treatment program." Ramsay discussed the situation with Labby and they both believed it would be preferable for the clinics to take on the disease management work, and they had no doubt the clinics could handle it quite well. With a green light from CEO Dave Ford, Ramsay "went to all clinics and asked, 'Do you think you can meet all these DM requirements' and all five organizations said, 'Absolutely, this is the work we want to be doing.'"

CareOregon selected diabetes and depression, widespread among the plan's population, as the two diseases to focus the disease management efforts on. NCQA accreditation required intensive focus on two chronic conditions, with rigorous performance standards. Ramsay worked to teach and coach personnel at the five clinics on treatments for both depression and diabetes. She went to Seattle to get advanced training on how to implement the IMPACT model of depression care, which had been developed at the University of Washington and was widely considered to be a reliable, evidence-based approach to treating depression in a primary care setting. After her own training she returned to Portland and in turn trained personnel in the five clinics on how to apply the method. In addition, she brought in a trainer from the University of Washington for an intensive two-day training session for the clinics. The model requires that primary care personnel consult with a psychiatrist weekly to seek guidance on treating specific patients. Because most of the clinics did not employ a psychiatrist, CareOregon retained three psychiatrists to provide consultations with primary care teams.

There was no comparable model for diabetes, although there were a number of effective approaches in use in different parts of the country. One of those was being used at Group Health in Seattle, and Ramsay invited several experts from that organization to come to Portland to train the clinical teams in diabetes care. "One of the most encouraging results of this work on disease management has been the excitement and engagement of the nurses and care managers," says Ramsay. "They are so happy to be doing the meaningful work that they are uniquely positioned and trained to do. In order to be able to meet the NCQA disease management requirements, each clinic system had to make tough changes in its operations so that much of the nonclinical work nurses had been doing could be removed [and the nurses could instead] focus on this patient-centered clinical work. This was not easy, but they did it!" In January 2011, CareOregon earned its NCQA accreditation.

## Paying Providers Differently

The issue of how CareOregon would compensate its provider partners was pivotal. CareOregon was asking providers to do things—working in teams and managing populations—that were not reimbursable in a fee-for-service arrangement. "When we were at Southcentral, someone said, 'If we're going to do this you're going to have to pay us differently, right?'" says Labby. "We said, 'of course.' But neither they nor we had any idea at that point what it would look like. It was an open commitment."

The first iteration of a revised payment model had CareOregon paying providers bonuses for three elements: active participation in the collaborative (joining in the learning community, participating in meetings, submitting data, and so forth); quality improvement on diabetes, hypertension, and preventive screening (a 3 percent improvement in the quarterly metrics would yield a certain bonus, and a 5 percent improvement would result in a larger payment); and decline in utilization. But then things got trickier. An essential issue was how to define a provider group's panel of patients. Debra Read says this required answering such questions as, "Who was considered an active patient?" and, "What population do we measure? Is it the patients you've seen during the past three years? The past twenty-four months?"

The collaborative formed the data and reporting work group, with the data specialists from each provider organization convening with Read to work on these issues. There were frustrating early glitches and growing pains. Read says, for example, that early on "one clinic reported that they had more people eighteen and over than they had twelve and over, which was obviously impossible. It was a learning process." The data and reporting issues presented a vexing problem, "a whole new competence that primary care now has to have," Labby says. "It's outcomes-driven medicine. You need to look at population data and make sense of it." For example, after much discussion—some of it rather intense—the collaborative agreed that a patient would be defined as someone who had been seen in the clinic during the past twelve months.

This payment iteration started in 2009 and at the end of that year all provider groups were paid for participating and all had succeeded in improving measurable quality. Little progress, however, had been made in decreasing utilization. In the second year, 2010, the payment arrangement progressed. There would no longer be a payment merely for participating, but there would be payments for improvements on additional quality metrics, including access. The CareOregon team also realized that payments needed to recognize the differences among the clinics and adapt to those. For example, a clinic with a large migrant population had very few patients with diabetes. Thus it made no sense to provide an incentive at that clinic for something that was not a major population issue. More sensible was a bonus payment for quality improvement in immunizations and preventive care for children in that clinic. At the end of the second year there were further quality improvements as well as improvements in access and—this was a breakthrough—significant progress on decreasing hospital utilization.

## Results

By the end of 2011, Labby reports, all five clinics had spread the Primary Care Renewal model, with the result that seventy primary care teams in eighteen clinical locations had fully integrated the model into their daily work (Figure 3.1).

A study reported by Martha Hostetter (2011) found that the new model used by the clinical teams in the collaborative "has resulted in increased access, greater productivity, and improved care." The study, which focused on one of the collaborative partners (Legacy Clinic Emanuel), noted the importance of "building interdisciplinary care teams—with greater roles for nurse practitioners, nurses, medical assistants, social workers, receptionists, and other support staff." In 2011, David Labby, Debra Read, and Aaron Winkel wrote a paper in which they reported results from the work of the collaborative, and their analysis showed that "since 2007, hospitalizations and cost trends for CareOregon members assigned to the participating clinics have

**Figure 3.1. Primary Care Renewal: Patient-Centered Medical Home**

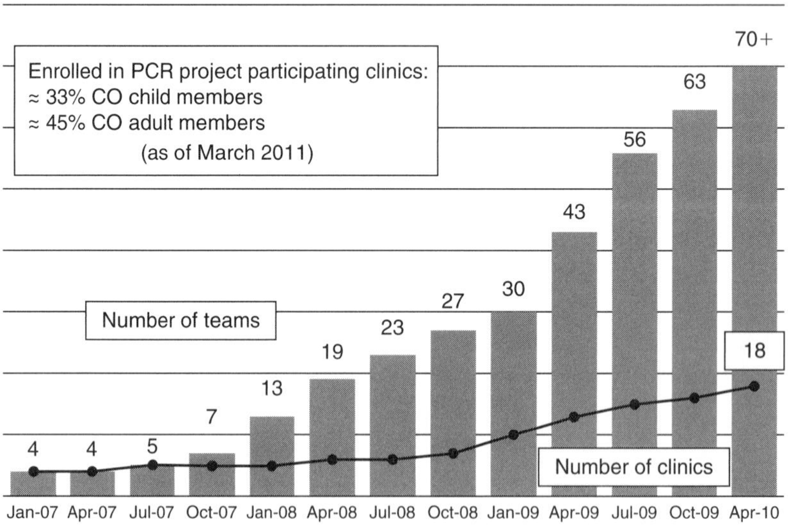

*Source:* CareOregon.

significantly declined; that markers of good clinical care, such as diabetes or hypertension control, have steadily increased; and that patients increasingly perceive that the clinics are meeting their individual needs."

Overall, the system redesign work resulted in a

- Decrease in ED and urgent care use of over 40 percent
- Decrease in specialty care use of over 50 percent
- Decrease in primary care visits of 20 percent
- Decrease in admissions and inpatient days of 30 percent

On the issue of cost, the paper reports that a dramatic shift has occurred in the cost of care for Medicaid patients in Primary Care Renewal clinics as compared with patients in other clinics. "Historically, the costs for the higher risk members in PCR clinics were significantly greater than for those in non PCR clinics . . . [due to the higher average risk scores]. Subsequent to the implementation of PCR, that pattern has now reversed—with total cost for the higher risk member population in the PCR clinics decreasing to . . . [the level] for non-PCR clinic members."

One of the most encouraging results of the new approach has been the avoidance of unnecessary and extremely expensive admissions and ED use. The data in Figures 3.2 and 3.3 get directly at the Triple Aim goal of cutting costs where appropriate.

Emergency department utilization increases in particular have played a significant role in Medicaid cost increases. In the time period after PCR implementation, the median ED visit rate for adult Medicaid patients in non-PRC clinics increased by 10 percent whereas emergency department rates among adult Medicaid patients in PRC clinics remained steady. As much as any fact, this is suggestive of the success Primary Care Renewal clinics have had in creating an authentic medical home for patients.

In Multnomah County, Kirchoff says Primary Care Renewal has resulted in better access for patients, essentially eliminating days of waiting by providing same-day appointments. It has cut the number of days to the next available appointment from four in February 2009 to one in February 2011. It has achieved significant improvements in patient surveys on key indicators such as the diabetes bundle as well as behavioral health. Patients now see their own

# Figure 3.2. Medicaid Adults: Inpatient (IP) Rates

IP stay rates for members in non-PCR clinics remained stable; during same time period, IP rates for non-PCR clinic members decreased significantly.

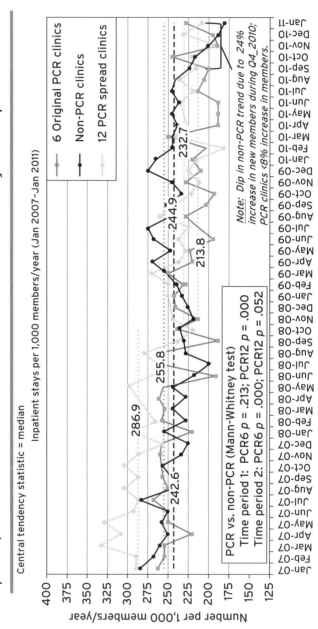

Central tendency statistic = median

Inpatient stays per 1,000 members/year (Jan 2007–Jan 2011)

- 6 Original PCR clinics
- Non-PCR clinics
- 12 PCR spread clinics

PCR vs. non-PCR (Mann-Whitney test)
Time period 1: PCR6 $p$ = .213; PCR12 $p$ = .000
Time period 2: PCR6 $p$ = .000; PCR12 $p$ = .052

Note: Dip in non-PCR trend due to 24% increase in new members during Q4_2010; PCR clinics <8% increase in members.

286.9   255.8   242.6   244.9   232.7   213.8

Number per 1,000 members/year

Source: Labby, Read, & Winkel, 2011.

**Figure 3.3. Medicaid Adults: Emergency Department Visit Rates**

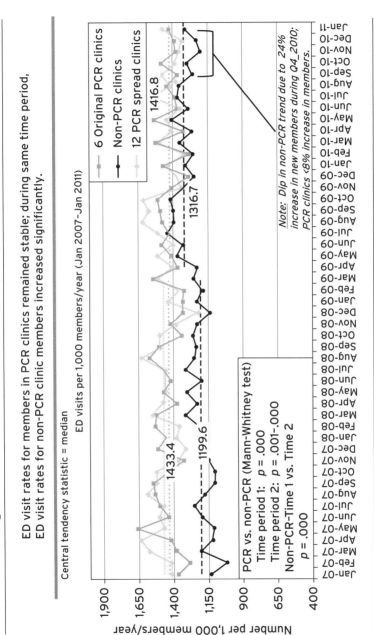

ED visit rates for members in PCR clinics remained stable; during same time period,
ED visit rates for non-PCR clinic members increased significantly.

Central tendency statistic = median

ED visits per 1,000 members/year (Jan 2007–Jan 2011)

Legend:
- 6 Original PCR clinics
- Non-PCR clinics
- 12 PCR spread clinics

1416.8
1316.7
1433.4
1199.6

PCR vs. non-PCR (Mann-Whitney test)
Time period 1:  p = .000
Time period 2:  p = .001-.000
Non-PCR-Time 1 vs. Time 2
p = .000

Note: Dip in non-PCR trend due to 24% increase in new members during Q4_2010; PCR clinics <8% increase in members.

Number per 1,000 members/year

*Source:* Labby, Read, & Winkel, 2011.

provider more than 85 percent of the time compared to about half that often before the new program. There has been a 13 percent improvement in patients who say they always get appointments as soon as they think they need them and a 13 percent improvement in those who say they always easily reach a member of their primary care team by phone when they need to. The county has achieved a 17 percent reduction in the incoming telephone call abandonment rate, an improvement sustained for a year so far, following this clinic's first attempt at a lean rapid improvement event.

On top of that, says Kirchoff, is something not particularly measurable: staff people from the clinics are telling her that "our patients are getting better care in our clinics than our employees get from their providers."

The data in Figures 3.4 and 3.5 demonstrate two of the ways in which PCR patients are reaping benefits from the new

**Figure 3.4. Chronic Disease Management Early Results: Percentage of Patients with Depression with 50 Percent Reduction in PHQ-9**

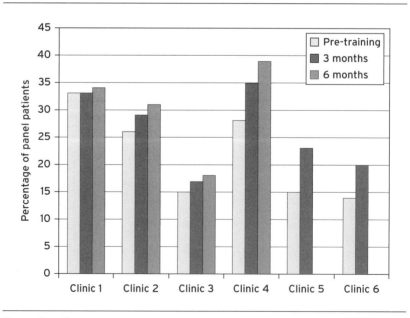

*Source:* CareOregon.

**Figure 3.5.  Chronic Disease Management Early Results:
Percentage of Patients with Diabetes Mellitus Meeting D3 Bundle**

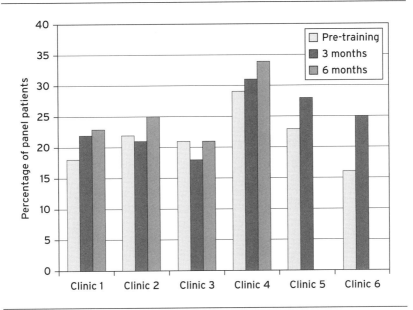

*Source:* CareOregon.
*Note:* The three elements in the D3 bundle are HbA1c < 8, LDL (low-density lipoprotein) < 100, and blood pressure under 130/80.

approach. They display improvement in disease-specific clinical indicators at a population level for depression and diabetes. These are clinical indicators that the CareOregon and clinic teams hoped would improve as a result of Primary Care Renewal and disease management.

Figures 3.6 and 3.7 indicate the steady improvement that has been occurring on the two key metrics of HbA1c screening for cases of diabetes and depression screening. The six clinics for which data are displayed are all in the same federally qualified health center, serving over 60 percent of the CareOregon adult members (Medicaid & dual eligibles) enrolled in the PCR initiative; they serve an urban area population with comparatively high acuity and high psychosocial comorbidity.

# Figure 3.6. Percentage of Patients with Diabetes with HbA1c Levels < 8 in the Past Six Months

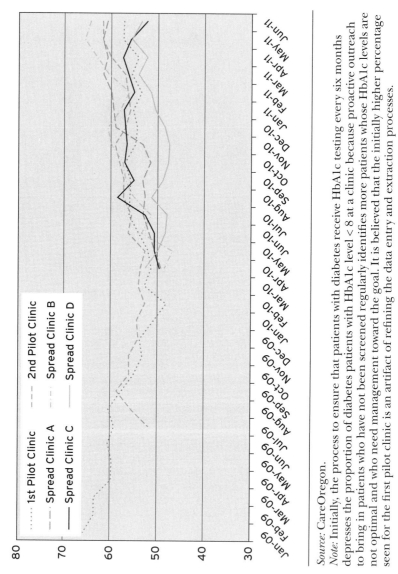

*Source:* CareOregon.

*Note:* Initially, the process to ensure that patients with diabetes receive HbA1c testing every six months depresses the proportion of diabetes patients with HbA1c level < 8 at a clinic because proactive outreach to bring in patients who have not been screened regularly identifies more patients whose HbA1c levels are not optimal and who need management toward the goal. It is believed that the initially higher percentage seen for the first pilot clinic is an artifact of refining the data entry and extraction processes.

# Figure 3.7. Percentage of Patients Eighteen Years and Older Screened for Depression in the Past Twelve Months

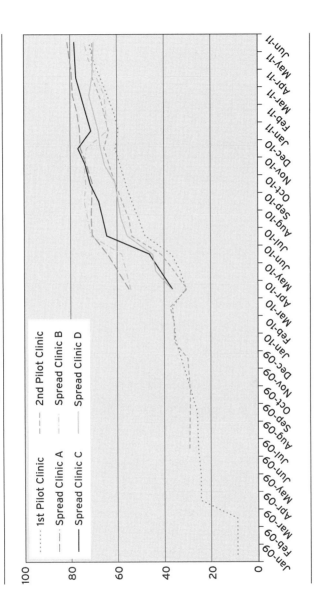

*Source:* CareOregon.

*Note:* This depression screening chart exemplifies what happened when some clinics piloted a new process and then it spread to other clinics. After the initial spread work was done, increasing the proportion of adults screened became the organization-wide focus of quality improvement work for several quarters.

### Figure 3.8. Survey of Health Care Providers at PCR Medical Home Model Clinics, 2009 and 2011

"I would recommend the PCR team-based approach to delivering proactive, comprehensive, patient-centered medical home care to my professional colleagues."

|  | Disagree/ Strongly Disagree | Neutral | Agree/ Strongly Agree | Total |
|---|---|---|---|---|
| Jan-Feb 2011—All PCR clinics | 4% | 9% | 87% | 100% |
| Nov 2009—6 original PCR clinics | 5% | 12% | 83% | 100% |
| Nov 2009—PCR spread clinics | 6% | 24% | 70% | 100% |

*Pioneer clinics* = Engaged in PCR medical home project for at least 1 ½ – 2 years.    *Spread clinics* = New clinics engaged in PCR medical home project for less than 12 months.

*Source:* CareOregon.

Finally, while all of this work has been going on, it is true that many providers have felt extra pressure to improve. But it is also true that the Primary Care Renewal approach has brought a high level of satisfaction to providers (Figure 3.8).

## Social Care

CareOregon CEO Dave Ford takes the long view. Going forward, he aspires to accelerate the work he and his colleagues are doing and to take it outside the walls of CareOregon's clinical collaborators. "The only way to outrun the bear is to invest forward in social infrastructure," he says—to begin to affect all those social determinants of health. He is particularly interested in a deeper engagement with young people in schools, with the hope of heading off problems before they develop. "We need to think about how [to] deal with so many social determinants and not simply improving the quality of the medical system," he says. "[Our work] has to be much more broadly about health drivers that exist in a person's life. That's the edge we stand on now."

This thinking is ambitious and may sound like a reach. But it was surely ambitious and a reach for CareOregon, a small health plan with very little market clout, to engage the Portland community in transforming care delivery to the city's neediest population. That transformative journey is still far from perfect or complete, but an important start has been made.

## Keys to Doing This Work

The members of the CareOregon leadership team are clear minded about the key ingredients needed for the work they are doing:

- **Leadership.** Capable and visionary leadership is required at every step.
- **Risk tolerance.** Everyone participating in a new approach needs to have some willingness to take risks in order to learn and improve.
- **A long-term view.** In order to protect the patient population, leaders need to constantly ask, "What is our long-term interest?"
- **Data competence.** The ability to gather needed data and to report them accurately must be pushed down to the clinical level.
- **Training competence.** The organization needs to possess or acquire the knowledge of how to carry out improvement, and it needs to teach these processes at the clinical level.
- **Visiting.** When moving from the status quo to a transformational model, seeing the changes can help to build will and stimulate breakthrough ideas.
- **Funding.** A source of funds to support the experimentation and improvement processes is essential.

# 4

# The Alternative Quality Contract

## A Payment Method Supporting the Triple Aim

An emerging consensus in the United States suggests that the traditional fee-for-service method of paying for health care is inadequate for the challenges of today and that the nation needs an approach that aligns provider payments with both the health of individual patients and the well-being of larger populations.

At the same time, a growing consensus among health care stakeholders focuses on the pursuit of value in health care—another way of characterizing the pursuit of the Triple Aim. Michael Porter, Elizabeth Teisberg, and Scott Wallace (2008) of the Harvard Business School say it's about value: "Value means the health outcomes achieved for the money spent." They add that "the best way truly to reduce health care cost is to improve its quality—better diagnoses, more timely treatment, less invasive methods, getting the right treatment to the right patient, fewer complications, and so on. Quality, defined in terms of outcomes, is the secret to success in health care."

In this chapter we write about an innovative contract that is aligned around quality. The Alternative Quality Contract (AQC) is a risk-based, capitated contract that provides global payments and significant bonuses for quality. It was created by a team at Blue Cross Blue Shield of Massachusetts and is now used by twelve provider organizations in that state, covering approximately 615,000 members (about two-thirds of the company's Massachusetts HMO membership).

Our focus here is on the experiences of two of these provider groups with the new contract. One group is a collaboration between Mount Auburn Hospital, a midsized facility in Cambridge, Massachusetts, and its affiliated independent physician organization. The other is Atrius Health, an alliance of medical groups comprising about eight hundred physicians, located in eastern Massachusetts.

At its core the Alternative Quality Contract is focused on the Triple Aim. It includes robust incentives to improve the individual quality of care for patients as well as the overall health of a defined population. And it contains powerful mechanisms to control costs. Researchers at the Harvard Medical School reported in 2011 that the Alternative Quality Contract "lowered medical spending while improving the quality of patient care relative to the traditional fee-for-service system." Michael E. Chernew, the study's senior author, observed that "the finding of reduced spending, together with improved quality in year-one of the contract, is significant. For policymakers contemplating improved payment models for US health care, reducing medical spending while improving quality and outcomes is the Holy Grail. While much remains to be seen over the next years of these AQC contracts and as the model expands to other providers, these early results provide reason for optimism" (Blue Cross Blue Shield of Massachusetts, 2011).

## Pay for Quality Not Quantity

In 2008, the leaders at Blue Cross Blue Shield of Massachusetts (BCBSMA), believing that perverse incentives built into the prevailing fee-for-service payment system led to waste and inefficiency, determined that instead of paying for procedures and volume, they wanted to pay for quality. They wanted a system that aligned the best interests of patients' health with what doctors and hospitals were paid to do. If they created a contract that provided incentives for quality and safety, would it lead to better outcomes, less waste, and more efficient use of health care dollars? They believed it would.

Blue Cross was certainly not alone in its viewpoint. Innovative provider organizations in Massachusetts and beyond had come to a similar view on their own. Leaders at organizations such as Atrius Health, for example, ardently supported global payments instead of fee-for-service, in the interest of population health. And it was clear that the national environment was ripe for such an approach. It seemed everywhere one looked during 2008 and 2009, another credible person or organization was saying that the United States needed to alter the health care payment system to pay for quality rather than volume. The waste and inefficiency fee-for-service produced was rapidly being revealed as was its failure to offer incentives for quality care. Under fee-for-service contracts, providers are paid for the volume of their work. One of the obvious and well-documented unintended consequences is what the Institute of Medicine identified as "overuse" of health care services. This unnecessary use is marbled throughout the system and costs Americans tens of billions of dollars annually. Another unintended consequence is that most of the things doctors can do to head off disease and keep their patients healthy are compensated only at very low rates or not at all under fee-for-service.

Neither private payers nor the government have typically been compensating physicians for improving the quality of health and life of patients with diabetes or those with any number of other chronic conditions.

Solving this problem presents one of the great and essential challenges in health care today and many excellent minds have sought a solution. There are alternative payment systems out there of course. The Geisinger Health Plan *bundled payment* model—ProvenCare—has received a great deal of positive attention. Initiated in 2006, the method sets a single price for coronary artery bypass grafting and hip replacement surgeries. In both cases the single fee covers all care related to the surgery—hospital and doctors' fees—including any readmissions necessary within ninety days of surgery. The bundled model is also sometimes called a *case rate* or an *episode-based payment*. The Geisinger approach creates a powerful inducement for providers to get the surgery right the first time because any complications or readmissions take a significant bite out of their bottom line. Thus quality care for the patient and financial success for the provider are well aligned.

The *Prometheus Payment* model has also received a fair amount of attention. It too involves payment for a bundle of services. "At its core, the Prometheus Payment model centers on packaging payment around a comprehensive episode of medical care that covers *all* patient services related to a single illness or condition," according to the Robert Wood Johnson Foundation, which supports the Prometheus work (Robert Wood Johnson Foundation, 2011). The plan provides financial incentives for clinical collaboration and for avoiding complications.

But fee-for-service remains the undisputed king of U.S. payment systems and that means the financial incentive for doctors is to do more—more office visits, more tests, more procedures—more of everything. Under fee-for-service there is little if any incentive to limit unnecessary tests and procedures, little if any incentive to provide the kind of financial stewardship that improves efficiency and eliminates waste.

The timing of Blue Cross's search for an alternative payment model was fortuitous. Throughout the health care reform debate in Washington, D.C., at that time, a series of scholars, practitioners, and policymakers echoed the same themes concerning fee-for-service and its misaligned incentives. Health economist Len Nichols (2010) wrote in the *New England Journal of Medicine* that "payment reform that rewards quality over volume is the key to using market forces to align incentives for patients, providers, and payers while reducing cost growth for taxpayers." Support for a payment system shift came from the Commonwealth Fund, the Institute for Healthcare Improvement (IHI), and other leading organizations. President Barack Obama said health care payments should be made "on the basis of improved quality as opposed to simply how many procedures you're doing."

## A Time for Action

In the winter of 2007, a team of a dozen-plus Blue Cross leaders convened in a windowless basement conference room (known as the Cave) working to come up with a plan. Collectively, the Cave team members possessed significant experience not only managing a health plan but also working for provider organizations, for consulting firms, and in academia. The team had extensive experience engaging with a diverse group of thinkers about where health care was headed and should go. Indeed, this was a pocket of Blue Cross that had a sort of think tank feel to it.

The Cave team members began by raising and dismissing the idea of a capitated contract, yet within forty-eight hours, they had returned to the notion. They focused on including rewards not only for efficiency but also for measurable improvement in quality on a specific list of metrics related to clearly improved patient health. The Cave team consensus was that the contract should send a clear message: if you improve the quality of patients' health, Blue Cross will reward you with significant bonus payments. The team's mantra at the time was that the contract "pays for quality/appropriateness rather than volume, complexity and intensity."

If the contract were to succeed, it would alter the relationship between physician groups and hospitals, turning them into business and clinical partnerships; it would also alter the relationship between the health plan and provider organizations because, at least in theory, the insurance company and providers would share goals of improved patient care and efficiency; it would result in more patient referrals to the lower-priced yet high-quality alternatives to the highest-priced tertiary hospitals (often those with iconic reputations); and it would seek to reduce unwarranted practice pattern variation and result in more evidence-based care.

Central to the contract was a strict limitation on the increase of capitated payments over time. This was critically important for it provided a powerful incentive for providers to curb their spending over the five-year life of the contract in order to remain in the black. "While the quality dollars were more than ever before, the real money was in the potential savings from increasing efficiency in global care," says Kate Koplan, MD, Atrius Health director of medical management.

Success would be measured by whether the contract bent the cost curve. From 2008 to 2009, medical spending by provider organizations with Blue Cross Blue Shield of Massachusetts contracts had grown nearly 12 percent on average. The explicit goal of the new Blue Cross approach was to cut that figure in half over the five-year period of the contract.

## Integrated Care

In a matter of a few weeks the Cave team generated the outlines of what it called the Alternative Quality Contract. The AQC encouraged provider organizations to behave in an integrated fashion—for physician groups and hospitals to work together under the contract as a combined entity that would take responsibility for cost and quality "across the continuum of care" for both inpatients and ambulatory patients. The contract's five-year term was designed to enable integrated systems to work together and refine their approaches through the years to produce progressively better results on quality and cost.

The contract established three ways in which provider organizations would be paid. First, they would receive a global payment designed to cover all medical services for a defined population of patients (adjusted for age, sex, and health status). This global payment was essentially a budget for all services received by a patient, including primary, specialty, and hospital care and pharmacy services.

Second, providers would receive additional payments over the term of the contract based on the annual rate of inflation as determined by the Consumer Price Index, which has been rising at a rate that is half or less of the rate of medical inflation. Blue Cross executives expected that this provision would play a key role in the contract's ability to bend the health care cost curve.

And third, providers could earn substantial bonus payments—up to 10 percent of the total contract—based on their performance on the quality metrics, both for ambulatory and for hospital-based patients. Bonus payments depended on which of the five ascending quality benchmarks (or *gates*) providers reached. The incentive payments, Blue Cross officials said at the time, were designed to "support providers in achieving the highest levels of safe, affordable, effective, patient-centered care."

Under the contract, providers would share risk with Blue Cross. Although some provider organizations in Massachusetts had a good deal of experience with risk-based contracts, many did not. Thus the amount of risk involved was unsettling to some providers. Recognizing this, Blue Cross put in place several ways to mitigate provider risk. Budgets would be adjusted annually based on shifts in the patient population's health status. Providers could choose to take on all the risk or they could take on any amount down to 50 percent, with the rest of the risk shared by Blue Cross. And reinsurance was required for all groups working under the contract, to protect them against particularly high claims.

Providers could also make money—potentially a great deal of money, as Dr. Koplan noted—from another contract element. If a provider organization was able to improve its efficiency and deliver care for less than the cost of its global budget, it could keep the budgeted funds (or share them with Blue Cross in those instances where contract risk was shared). This was a powerful incentive to reduce waste in the delivery system. If the groups—through lean management or other techniques—could improve their efficiency and deliver care for less money than the budget allowed, there was a significant financial upside.

The Blue Cross team said that its goal over the five-year term of the contract was to cut the annual increase in health care costs in half. Team members believed that this would make premium increases both more affordable and predictable.

Provider organizations seeking to work within an AQC could be large multispecialty groups or collaborations between a hospital and independent physician organization. This type of contract could also cover independent collections of small physician practices. Whatever its structure, the covered group would have to have a strong primary care base, with a minimum of 5,000 Blue Cross HMO members or point-of-service plan members. (This restriction effectively limited ACQ participation to plans in which plan members are required to have a designated primary care physician.)

## Performance Measures: The Foundation of the Contract

The quality metrics Blue Cross proposed were compiled by Dana Gelb Safran, senior vice president for performance measurement and improvement at the company, using input from community and academic experts. The metrics would be subject to intense discussion with provider groups in the months to come and they would shift somewhat, but just about all the metrics Safran originally proposed became essential elements in the contract. In an interview with the Commonwealth Fund, Safran explained the metrics:

> Every group participating in the AQC has the same set of performance incentives and measures. The measure set draws entirely from well-validated, clinically important, nationally accepted measures of clinical processes, clinical outcomes, and patient experiences and encompasses both ambulatory and inpatient care. Prior to launching the first contracts, we met with early adopters [of the contract] to get detailed input on the proposed measure set. This led to some minor adjustments, but these provider organizations agreed that the measures we had chosen were fair, important, and clinically appropriate.
>
> For every measure, there are fixed performance targets—"gates"— that do not change over the five-year contract and are the same for every AQC organization. For each measure, Gate 1 represents the score that constitutes the beginning of good performance— performance that we think is worthy of additional financial recognition. Gate 5 is an empirically derived score that represents the outer limit of what can be reliably achieved on the measure. A group that achieves Gate 5 across the whole set of measures, which is a very difficult task, earns an additional 10 percent on the global budget. Those whose performance on the measure set is at Gate 1 earn an additional 2 percent. Between Gates 1 and 5, incentive payments increase in a way that motivates improvement

on the early and middle part of that continuum, with less emphasis on getting from Gate 4 to Gate 5. This structure has allowed us to reward both good performance and performance improvement—an important feature of the model that helps to refute a widely held belief that one has to choose between rewarding performance or rewarding improvement [Commonwealth Fund, 2010a].

There were more process than outcomes measures, but, because of their clinical importance, the weighting was heavily tilted toward outcomes measures. Measures such as blood pressure control in the ambulatory setting, for example, were given three times the weight of a process measure. The groups covered by the AQC would make these measures the subjects of intense focus, for these were the metrics with the greatest potential for improvement.

Here in brief are the areas addressed by the Blue Cross quality metrics (Commonwealth Fund, 2010a):

### Hospital Quality and Safety
#### Clinical Process Measures

- Acute MI (acute myocardial infarction [AMI]) care elements that must not be omitted and care elements that need to be performed within a defined period of time
- Heart failure care
- Pneumonia care
- Surgical care

#### Clinical Outcomes Measures

- Hospital-acquired infections
- Complications after major surgery (AMI, PE/DVT [pulmonary embolism/deep vein thrombosis], pneumonia)
- Obstetric trauma

#### Patient Care Experiences

- Communication quality: physicians
- Communication quality: nurses
- Responsiveness
- Discharge support/planning

### Ambulatory Care Quality
*Clinical Process Measures*

- Depression
- Diabetes
- Cardiovascular disease
- Cancer screening
- Pediatric: appropriate testing/treatment
- Pediatric: well child visits

*Clinical Outcomes Measures*

- Diabetes (HbA1c in poor control, LDL-C control, blood pressure control)
- Hypertension (blood pressure control)
- Cardiovascular disease (blood pressure control, LDL-C control)

*Patient Care Experiences*

- Communication quality
- Whole-person orientation/knowledge of patients
- Integration of care
- Access to care

## Clinical Practice Pattern Variation

Dana Safran had studied large quantities of data and found that in eastern Massachusetts extensive and widespread clinical practice pattern variation presented a major obstacle to improving the quality of care and controlling costs. After finding that physicians in the same practice treated a particular condition in many different ways, she concluded that even though some of those treatments might have been effective, the variation was so great that "they can't all be right." In her research Safran found wide variation in the treatment of a broad array of conditions, including hypertension, depression, migraine headaches, arthritis, low back pain, and much more. One of the key elements of the AQC, she believed, was that as clinicians focused on improving their quality scores, unexplained variation would quickly emerge. And once it was clear and out in the open in a clinical practice, she was confident that clinicians would move to narrow the gap and move toward standardized best practices. Otherwise it would be exceedingly difficult to improve quality scores. Thus Blue Cross made it a priority to package claims data for providers in ways that highlighted variation, emphasizing unexplained clinical practice pattern variation.

## *Not* the Capitation of Old

On the surface the contract was a capitated arrangement that the Blue Cross officials knew would give some people in health care flashbacks to the ugly days of managed care in the 1990s. But this new approach was quite different, and Blue Cross took pains to make that amply clear, emphasizing that during the '90s capitated arrangements seemed too often focused more on money than quality of care and that the metrics did not exist at the time to do the sort of quality measurement possible now.

Jeanette Clough, CEO at Mount Auburn Hospital, saw right away that the AQC was quite different from the payment models used in the "bad old days of capitation." "This wasn't cut, cut, cut," she says. "It was improve care and get a reward." The old capitated models focused on cutting the cost of care, and in many cases there was fear that important care was withheld to meet a financial goal. But Clough and other leaders were acutely aware of the shortcomings of the earlier capitated model and they also knew that under the AQC they would report on quality measures that would reveal any withholding of services from patients. Such withholding, if it were to occur, would result in penalties to the provider. And the way the contract was structured, withholding services would in fact be counterproductive. If a provider group withheld important care from patients to meet a budget, that would be revealed by the group's failures to meet or improve on quality metrics.

Blue Cross's new proposal sought to create an incentive for providers to do as much as they possibly could to keep patients healthy, for it was in doing so that they would reap the greatest financial reward.

Yet the AQC was not an easy sell. Many provider organizations, fearing financial losses under the contract, were reluctant to take it on. Others doing well financially under fee-for-service arrangements wanted no part of such an experiment. But there were also leaders of provider organizations who believed health care in the United States was headed in a new direction. For the most part these were organizations that looked ahead and saw health care moving toward a post-fee-for-service world where accountable care organizations or other innovative models might emerge as powerful players and thus where integration mattered.

## Mount Auburn Hospital and Affiliated Physicians

Notwithstanding some suspicion and a certain level of resistance from providers, the first group to sign on for the AQC did so with enthusiasm. The ideal arrangement for the contract was an integrated health system or a collaborative effort between a hospital and physician group. Mount Auburn Hospital in Cambridge joined together with an independent physicians group affiliated with the hospital, the Mount Auburn Cambridge Independent Practice Association (MACIPA), and engaged in serious discussions about accepting the AQC.

CEO Jeanette Clough formed a leadership team with Drs. Barbara Spivak and Robert Janett, the president and medical director, respectively, of MACIPA. MACIPA comprised five hundred physicians on staff at Mount Auburn Hospital and the Cambridge Health Alliance. This hospital and physician group team held a series of intense discussions with representatives from Blue Cross, going through the details of the contract. Clough knew she held some strong cards. She was aware that Blue Cross was having a difficult time selling the new contract to providers and she was more than willing to use that leverage to get a better deal as the first adopter of the contract (that deal included a bonus payment to Mount Auburn–MACIPA for being the first provider organization to adopt the contract).

The contract appealed to Clough and her team for many reasons. One was that Mount Auburn had years of experience managing risk contracts and was quite comfortable doing so. The major reason, however, was that Mount Auburn was on a mission to improve the quality and efficiency of care to its patients, and the AQC provided the kind of framework that would enable it to do that. One of the most appealing aspects of the contract was that it would leave the great majority of decisions about patient care up to doctors. There would be Blue Cross policy and coverage parameters, of course, but the traditional role of the insurer peering over the physician's shoulder would be much less intrusive under this contract.

## Agreeing on the Metrics

The most difficult part of the negotiation centered on exactly what metrics would be used to measure performance. This was, during the negotiation stage, the heart of the matter. "We spent about a year working to clarify exactly what the metrics were and how they would be measured," says Clough. "That was the toughest part. There were many questions: How to report the measures? Whose data would be used?" In the past Mount Auburn leaders had experienced difficult discussions with the government and private payers concerning measurement, and there was some worry on the Mount Auburn side that there would be disputes about the metrics going forward. "We were concerned," says Clough, "that half way through the contract they'd say, 'Well, we didn't mean *that*,' or, 'We wanted you to measure it *this* way.' We needed black-and-white clarity about the quality metrics—*exactly* what we would report."

At the end of the discussion the two sides agreed to use claims data collected by Blue Cross that would then be reviewed and validated at Mount Auburn.

MACIPA president Barbara Spivak believed the metrics chosen would be readily accepted by the MACIPA physicians. "These were things that were measurable and reasonable," she says. "For the hospital, to be honest, these were fairly standard CMS [Centers for Medicare & Medicaid Services] measures and not all that controversial. On the ambulatory side, HEDIS [Healthcare Effectiveness Data and Information Set] is a nationally accepted standard, so you have to accept that. And there aren't other great standards out there for quality."

When Spivak looked at the ambulatory metrics she saw that MACIPA doctors weren't doing badly on them but clearly also had room for improvement. "At first it was intimidating to me as medical director," says Rob Janett. "It was mind boggling. Where do we begin? We began with data so we knew where our strengths and weakness were. And we started with important diseases to capture the attention of our physicians. We wanted to start by working on issues where there was broad consensus about clinical goals and desired outcomes."

Chronic conditions were an obvious starting point given their prevalence and enormous expense for the health care system. Also, even though there were financial rewards for hitting the marks on process metrics, the rewards for achieving outcomes goals were triple that. For example, "if you measure glycosylated hemoglobin you get a certain reward, but if you achieve excellent glycemic control for a patient you get a reward that is a multiple of the process measure," Janett says. "Checking cholesterol levels gets you $X$ but achieving [an] LDL level less than 100 gets a multiple of $X$. That's really where the clinical goals lie—achieving control of the diabetes."

Once the Mount Auburn–MACIPA leadership team had worked through the agreement with Blue Cross, there remained the challenge of explaining and selling the contract to the MACIPA physicians. The MACIPA leaders "can only suggest, incentivize, teach, cajole," says Janett. "We use the powers of persuasion, peer pressure, education. We said to the doctors, 'Look, if we can improve according to these metrics we can predict that our financial position will improve and, more importantly, we'll be doing really good care for patients.'" Janett saw the AQC as a potentially powerful business asset, for he was confident that the MACIPA doctors could achieve measurable improvement on the metrics. Once they did so, the community would learn of their success and thus Mount Auburn would attract new patients and potentially better contracts with health plans. The MACIPA doctors got it quickly. Although concerned with the level of risk, they could see the potential.

Barbara Spivak says there were two other troublesome issues at the start. First was the reality that the contract sought to reduce the cost increases by half over five years. "People were very nervous about that concept," says Spivak. They worried about what would happen if there was a catastrophic epidemic of some sort or very expensive new cures for diseases. But she made the case that the health care environment in the country was changing rapidly and that "clearly people were beginning to talk about keeping health expense trends down and employers paying less and getting control on health care expenses."

In addition, she made the case to her doctors that Blue Cross was using the prior year's expense level to set the basis for the AQC budget going forward. Spivak and her physicians knew that under changed circumstances that budget was more than sufficient. She knew, for example, that far too many patients were going to expensive downtown hospitals and specialists for issues that could be handled at Mount Auburn. Under existing contracts the physicians had little incentive to keep those patients within the Mount Auburn system. Under the AQC, however, the incentives would be substantial and right away Spivak saw significant savings possibilities: "For a group like ours, where more than we would like was being done in expensive hospitals downtown, we knew that if we could move what could be done at Mount Auburn—and lot could be—it would be better for our docs because they would have the volume and better for Mount Auburn because they would have the volume and better for patients because there would be better coordination of care."

Ultimately the decision by the MACIPA physicians on whether to take on the Alternative Quality Contract came down to the fact that they believed this was the right way to reform health care—focusing on measurable improvement of their patients' health.

## Making the Contract Work

Rob Janett has worked as part of the MACIPA system for more than twenty years. Throughout those years, he says, many independent physician practices that make up MACIPA have worked to become ever more proficient at managing risk. This has always meant a careful eye on expenses. Thus the theory of the AQC was appealing from the start.

MACIPA's historical relationship with Blue Cross Blue Shield of Massachusetts might have posed an obstacle. "In earlier times Blue Cross was a very difficult company to deal with," says Janett.

Blue Cross had been too bureaucratic and sometimes too auto-cratic as well in the past, and there had been dealings that left a bad taste in the mouths of MACIPA doctors. Because MACIPA is a membership organization that serves essentially as a contractor on behalf of the organization—the doctors are independent and directly employed by neither Mount Auburn Hospital nor the MACIPA association—they could not be ordered what to do.

However, the attitude toward Blue Cross "changed with the AQC," says Janett. "It was a revolutionary moment in our relation-ship. We saw the potential right away and we wanted to be the first on board. We believed if we were first we could help them design a good program—one that would be beneficial to patients, doc-tors, and the health plan."

During the first year of the contract (2009), the hospital and the physicians worked on improving as many measures as they could take on at the start, and they quickly showed some prog-ress. An analysis of patients with difficult disease states and high costs resulted in clinicians focusing intently on this population.

Provider groups working under the AQC receive monthly reports from Blue Cross that mark their progress—whether they are on, ahead, or behind budget; whether utilization is up; and much more. Providers can see exactly how their budget money is being spent and can quickly identify areas of possible overuse—imaging tests or name brand drugs, for example—and work on that.

Knowing that a very small percentage of patients account for a high proportion of costs, MACIPA physicians use software to study their population, looking to identify members at great-est risk for a wide variety of health issues. Under the AQC, they believe that investing in this software is wise, given the potential return both financially and from finding and helping challeng-ing patients. They use the software to search through millions of lines of data to find patients who have gaps in care.

Once identified, these patients received significant atten-tion from high-risk case managers who reach out to patients and work to guide them to the appropriate care in the appropriate setting. Among the results of this, Janett believes, are a reduc-tion in the number of particularly frail patients calling 911 for a trip to the emergency department as well as fewer inpatient stays and avoidable return trips to the hospital. Getting the right care and prevention to patients before they get into trouble means better quality for the patients and less expense for MACIPA. For the reality is that when patients get into trouble because they have not had the care screenings and prevention they need, they are far more likely to wind up at the ED or as an inpatient. And those are costs borne directly by MACIPA physicians. "We work to make sure that there is a care plan in place for these patients so we can avoid having people fall through the cracks," says Janett. "We make sure there is a clear care plan in place so they have an alternative to calling 911 when they are sick or afraid. That way we can cut out some unneeded or duplicative services."

## Managing Outside Referrals

An essential element in making the AQC work is something that often goes against the grain of Americans' desire to have the freedom to go to any doctor or hospital they wish to go to. Under the AQC, they can do so, but the plan doesn't work very effectively if patients are constantly going outside the network for services. This has a huge impact on the cost of care. When patients need high-level tertiary care beyond the capability of Mount Auburn hospital, the MACIPA leadership asks doctors to refer selectively "to tertiary places that give us good value." That means not referring to some of the dominant players in the eastern Massachusetts marketplace and referring to others whose brands may be less well known but who nonetheless provide high-quality care at a lower cost.

The MACIPA physicians have made a significant effort to reduce referrals outside Mount Auburn and Cambridge hospitals. When patients remain within the Mount Auburn sphere, care is better coordinated and therefore, at least theoretically, safer. Handoffs and transitions go more smoothly. This has meant coaching primary care physicians on how to talk with patients about choosing a hospital for their care. Many patients come in with strong, preconceived notions about a particular brand name hospital—typically one of the large teaching facilities in downtown Boston. Perhaps they have been a patient there before or have had family members there. Or perhaps they are basing their preference, as is often the case, on reputation. This is somewhat tricky territory for doctors, but with coaching, MACIPA physicians have had success in talking patients through their choices.

"With a well-managed discussion, patients understand that there is a benefit to beginning at home," says Janett. "I tell my patients, 'I'd like you to try the doctor I know here best and whose skills I trust. I'd like you to talk with her. I think you'll be pleased. If you are not satisfied, talk with me again, and we will find you the best specialist for your problem.'" Janett tells patients that if they see a particular specialist he knows within the MACIPA system, the care will be well coordinated. He points out that he and the specialist use the same electronic medical record. Coordination of care between a primary care physician and a specialist is best within the MACIPA family, he says. "You don't win every one of those discussions," he says, "but if you engage the patient in a shared effort to try and deliver coordinated care of high value, most patients will at least try it and most patients will be satisfied."

Dr. Barbara Spivak, the MACIPA president, shares that view. "When I talk with a patient about it, one of the prime things I point out is that there is equally good quality at Mount Auburn" as compared with major Boston medical centers, she says. "But we have a coordination of care advantage. I can manage the care and help shepherd patients through something if they are at Mount Auburn. I can get easy information and I know the doctors and I am there. That sways a lot of people." Because she has to rely on a discharge summary rather than ongoing reports and personal knowledge, "it's much harder to manage the care when people . . . [are discharged] from another hospital."

By the end of 2010, an increasing volume of work that previously would have gone to larger downtown facilities was being done at Mount Auburn. And the majority of the cases that went to downtown hospitals did so appropriately, given that they were beyond the capability of the Mount Auburn facility.

Dr. Karen Boudreau, who was working at Blue Cross Blue Shield of Massachusetts when the Alternative Quality Contract was created, has studied payment reform options as medical director for the IHI Continuum Portfolio. Boudreau observes that at a basic level under fee-for-service, physicians don't pay much attention to whether a patient is going to a high-cost facility for care: "It doesn't matter to them whether a patient is in a nursing home or at home after knee surgery, even when there is no need for a patient to be anywhere other than home." This attitude, she says, adds significant costs to the health care system. "But when there is a global payment system, you manage those high costs, and you say it *does* matter to us where the patient is and that is the most appropriate place at the lowest cost. When you are accountable for the whole picture, you think about those things more broadly." She knows that there are people in health care who push back and say, "when you think about it more broadly you'll withhold care." But she doesn't agree that this is what happens: "I just don't buy it."

## Changing the Way Providers Think

Rob Janett says that among the most important challenges in the AQC journey is the need for altering the culture in provider organizations. This is a recurring theme found across the country whenever provider organizations seek to improve their systems of care. Doctors have traditionally been trained to work independently, with a maximum degree of autonomy, and moving to more standardized, evidence-based care is often seen as an infringement on that way of working.

Barbara Spivak agrees, stating in a Commonwealth Fund (2010b) case study: "Neither the physicians nor the hospitals like to be told what to do and how to do it. Doctors in particular are used to doing everything on their own. And the reality is that when you're starting an ACO you have to deal with people's anger and disappointment that the world is changing. And I believe the way to do that is to develop a team that's going to help them do what they want, which is give better care to their patients."

Spivak believed that if MACIPA was to be successful going forward its members would have to demonstrate an ability to manage care effectively across a population. "Practices do have to revamp themselves to do that," she says. "If you look at access, care management, shared decision making, electronic communications with patients—we really need to work with our docs to change their practices, absolutely." They would have to get better at going way beyond the visit, "not just dealing with the patient in front of you," says Spivak, "but dealing with *all* your patients with diabetes. We're asking our physicians to do lots more outreach than they have ever done before."

That initial hurdle was difficult enough, but the MACIPA leaders also faced a far more difficult challenge. "The other major issue in terms of culture change is helping to wean doctors from longstanding fee-for-service incentives and toxicity," Janett says. "It is very hard to change the way they think. If you are not going to order a test when it is a marginal call, you have to have a certain amount of confidence in yourself. If there is no good evidence one way or the other, you try and err on the side of a less expensive, less invasive approach before deciding to do a test or biopsy or procedure."

The shift in thinking and approach required of clinicians as they adapt to the AQC is not easy. "Under fee-for-service it is very comforting for doctors to know that if you do more you get paid more," observes Clough. "It's very hard to turn that on its head—'You mean I can make more by paying attention to quality? Managing patient's drugs? Managing patients on an outpatient side versus inpatient?' It's hard for people to make that kind of leap and still feel like they're going to be whole."

So how does culture change occur in this realm? The physician group's leaders relied on evidence. They showed the doctors, for example, that MACIPA rate of ordering biopsies for skin lesions was double the rate of other physician groups in Greater Boston. Change did not come overnight, but doctors were often persuaded by such evidence, and over time, MACIPA whittled away at the numbers of expensive, unnecessary tests.

But at what point was too much being asked of the physicians? How much change could they really handle? Going from a fee-for-service model to a global payment model shocked the provider system in many ways. "One of my biggest concerns is asking too much of our doctors," says Janett. "We're asking for a lot of change in the way they think and I am concerned about the possibility of change fatigue."

It is not as though the doctors weren't working hard before the AQC became a factor in their practice—they certainly were. In fact many were stressed and frazzled. In addition, they had had to adjust to the installation of a new system of electronic medical records—an event highly stressful and disturbing to a practice in and of itself. And then on top of that, they had to deal with all the foundational changes demanded by the AQC.

But the doctors have risen to the occasion by working in a more collaborative, team-based way. In Janett's own practice, for example, he now works more than he did before with care management teams—doctors, nurses, physician assistants, front desk staff, and others—combing through patient registries looking for those individuals needing key tests or screenings. An important benefit of this approach has been a sense of empowerment and increased energy among staff members. "They take pride in the outcomes at the end of the month when we see an improvement in the diabetes metric or colon cancer screening metric," says Janett. "It builds a lot of team spirit and pride. It gives people a lot more job satisfaction. People know that by reaching out to patients overdue for colon cancer screening they are saving lives."

## Handling Frustrations

There are, of course, plenty of frustrations to be dealt with under the new contract. For example, if Mount Auburn follows through on a certain metric—such as giving an aspirin to a cardiac patient—but that act goes unrecorded for some reason, then from a financial perspective it is as though it never happened. And the process of getting systems aligned to make sure that everything done was recorded had some bumpy moments.

Other frustrations include the relentless push in modern health care to purchase the latest and most expensive equipment—even when there is no tangible proof that it provides better quality care. There is significant consumer pressure for a facility to acquire the latest hardware, says Janett. He notes that increasing numbers of men undergoing prostate surgery prefer a robotic method, even though, says Janett, "it's not necessarily better. They want a robotic technique but we don't have a robot. As a result we've lost some business to more expensive facilities." Such marketplace forces eventually caused the Mount Auburn leadership to relent and purchase a robot. "You don't want to jump into expensive, unproven new technology just because it's there," says Janett, "but the expectations of patients are driving some of us to do that."

Spivak expresses concern about the sophisticated IT systems required to measure and track care and to improve care while keeping costs down. Systems providing high-quality, timely data are essential, she says. But she also notes that "building and maintaining these systems to improve care is expensive. How to sustain the payment structure for managing care will be a challenge in the future. Doctors certainly will not be willing to pay for . . . [such systems] out of their revenue stream unless the possibility of 'surplus' is worth it. Providers are certainly interested in improving care and have shown a willingness to work hard to do so. The question will be how to pay for the infrastructure."

## Getting Better Results

Two years into the AQC effort, the Mount Auburn–MACIPA collaboration has improved quality scores and financial results. And physicians are generally happy with the new approach to practicing and with "their financial rewards," says Janett. A sense of competition among the individual physicians and groups within MACIPA has helped to drive improvement on quality scores. Teamwork has paid off. Halfway through the term of the contract, MACIPA had achieved approximately 60 percent of its internal quality targets, which was greater progress at a faster rate than its leaders had expected.

Blue Cross data showed conclusively that during the contract's first two years, providers within the AQC improved their quality of care much faster than clinical groups that worked under another type of contract did.

"The AQC marries two ideas," says Janett. "One is full risk capitation. It puts you in the driver's seat and places responsibility with you to assure the care you deliver to patients is efficient." The other idea is using "quality metrics to guard against pitfalls of full risk capitation while making up for risks of fee-for-service. The AQC gets people focused on doing quality and [controlling] cost. And we are constraining the growth of cost. We're bending the trend. Our costs are going up slower than the trend around us."

Janett notes that the new approach demands a great deal of work. "This is not easy stuff," he says. "It requires a lot of work that is not compensated in a standard fee-for-service arrangement. There is a lot of work before and after a visit, on the telephone.

The old model of a doctor waiting for patients to come and see him is antiquated. It does not achieve the kind of reliable care we need." This new approach is "about working with people intensively on population management, not just patients coming to see you. You have to worry about every patient on your panel. You need to reach out to them."

Although Mount Auburn and MACIPA improved their scores in 2011 over 2010, there were some areas where they did not perform as well, and Spivak and her colleagues are conducting a root cause analysis to try to figure out why. And that raises an issue that is yet to be answered in the early stages of the AQC: How sustainable are the gains?

"Just because you did it one year doesn't mean you are done," says Spivak. "Just because a patient's A1c is in control in 2010 doesn't mean they don't go off the bandwagon in 2011. You have to continue, continue, continue to monitor everything." She cites variation as an example of a challenge to sustainability. "Sometimes a decrease in variation holds and other times it slips back. Unfortunately, more often than not it does slip back."

Although working under the AQC is challenging, it is also rewarding both financially and in terms of the quality of care. Janett clearly prefers the AQC to fee-for-service, in part because it affords him the freedom to "do what's right" for the patient but also because it eliminates the "toxic incentives" of fee-for-service; incentives that make a doctor's life a grind and don't align the patient's best interests with payment.

Clough is convinced that the AQC provides a model for others throughout the country. "I absolutely do think the AQC improves quality," she says, "and people recognize that. We're bombarded by people from different parts of the country wanting to know about AQC and how we do it. The AQC is a tremendous model and has really given us the opportunity—as I believed it would—to improve quality and control costs."

## Atrius Health

Atrius Health signed the Alternative Quality Contract in July 2009 (covering calendar year 2009), after working toward the AQC path in a transition contract. Atrius Health is the largest independent physician alliance organization in the state of Massachusetts, with one thousand doctors serving nearly one million patients through six multispecialty groups: Harvard Vanguard Medical Associates, Dedham Medical Associates, Granite Medical Group, South Shore Medical Center, Southboro Medical Group, and Reliant Medical Group (formerly Fallon Clinic).

Some of the Atrius Health groups—particularly Harvard Vanguard—had a long history of risk contracting, but the sheer size and scope of the AQC quality metrics and the financial implications were far beyond anything they had ever attempted before. All six groups under the Atrius umbrella had engaged in pay-for-performance contracts, but they were minuscule compared with the AQC. Typically these contracts had included one or two metrics—and rarely if ever more than three—with targets that were not particularly challenging. And the financial rewards for reaching those goals were not that significant either. Dr. Richard Lopez, chief medical officer at Atrius, found that the teams could manage those contracts fairly easily with limited resources. "The AQC was a very different type of animal," says Lopez, "because on the ambulatory outpatient side alone there were thirty-two metrics instead of one or two."

Also, the performance improvement targets were far more ambitious than any previously tackled by the Atrius groups. "The performance metrics were really stretch targets," Lopez says. "You had to be a top performer in eastern Massachusetts to achieve the maximum bonus and goals."

One important advantage was the five-year length of the contract. Atrius and other providers had found one-year, pay-for-performance contracts limiting in that by the time they had ramped up to implement changes, the contract period was well under way. With a five-year time frame Atrius leaders felt comfortable that they could take some time to plan, invest in, and implement changes, knowing that they would be measured against the same metrics for five years, that they would not be aiming at a moving target.

At the start clinical leaders at Atrius felt that targeting all the metrics for action was too much to do at once. They decided instead to focus for the first couple of years on their fifteen "top-tier" metrics, which related to diabetes, hypertension, and cardiovascular issues and included all AQC outcomes measures. Not all of the fifteen are AQC metrics, however, as Atrius thought it important from a public health perspective to include smoking and obesity-related measures as well.

The Atrius leaders decided to apply the AQC metrics in the care of all their patients, including those covered by insurance companies other than Blue Cross Blue Shield of Massachusetts. If they were applying the metrics only to Blue Cross patients, Blue Cross data would have sufficed. But because they were casting a much wider net, they needed good data on all Atrius patients—including patients covered by other insurance plans. Thus, relying solely on Blue Cross data would have made it impossible for Atrius to do comprehensive population management.

In addition, they did not believe their clinicians would be comfortable with treating Blue Cross patients differently from other patients. "We realized that our ability to report information the practices needed around quality and medical expense was really limited," says Lopez. "We would create an Excel file or a PDF and send it out in an e-mail, but it wasn't what . . . [the clinicians] wanted, and we realized we did not have the expertise in house to mine the data so that it was accessible and people could use it to manage patient care."

They knew they needed to provide data to twenty-one Atrius clinical sites throughout the region so that each site knew where it stood on the measures. But the data Blue Cross was providing were based on claims and took too long to process and distribute. Thus, the data was not as timely as what Lopez and his colleagues needed. Atrius needed timely data in a form that could be easily accessed and used by clinicians and other staff throughout its system to target areas for improvement. Atrius had previously built a rich data warehouse based on a vast store of information mined from the system's electronic medical records as well as certain claims data and that warehouse evolved over time.

## Developing Powerful Performance Data

"It started with simple registries of patients at the site level and with aggregated performance rates at the group level," says Lopez. "It expanded over time to include site-level performance and individual primary care physician performance. The sharing of the site- and physician-based metrics at the sites was a particularly helpful communication and motivation tool."

An Atrius team, led by Dr. Kate Koplan, the Atrius director of medical management, developed a separate database for all the variables required to report on the top-tier metrics; this helped to make reporting the metrics easier and more efficient. This database was called the "quality measurement data mart." Then the question arose of the best way to get information out to the various Atrius practice sites. Having used PDFs and Excel files without much success, Lopez and Koplan realized that they needed a more sophisticated distribution system, one that could provide reports on clinicians' desktops and allow physicians and other team members to drill down into the data for more specific information. Lopez says that this realization "highlighted a weakness in our information management. We had a great amount of data but had difficulty getting it out to users in a usable format."

A new director of analytics and reporting systems was hired to refine and develop the data warehouse and report distribution systems to better meet ongoing and future needs. Producing real-time information in a format that clinicians and other staff would actually use was a significant step. "We could know what blood pressure was yesterday for a panel and an individual, and which patients got their tests done and which didn't," says Lopez.

Because of the principle of applying the same level of care to all patients, regardless of insurance plan, none of the data sent out to clinical teams carried any identification of the insurance plan that any patient used. "All the insurance information is invisible" on the performance rosters, says Lopez. "Whether [a] Medicare fee-for-service patient or a Blue Cross Blue Shield of Massachusetts AQC patient, you get the same high level of care."

The performance data proved immensely powerful. The information went out monthly to the clinical teams throughout Atrius Health, comparing the performance of clinics, teams within clinics, and ultimately individual physicians. Internally, anyone could see whose panels were improving the most. "That helped tremendously," says Lopez, "because providers are driven by a desire to provide quality care to patients, but they are also very competitive, and . . . sharing performance data . . . really opens the eyes of many doctors and really helps spur improvement." One obvious result was that some physicians whose performance levels weren't particularly impressive sought out colleagues at the upper end to learn what they had done in terms of panel management.

Although the performance measures spurred physicians and their teams on to more concerted efforts with patients, a different data set guided those efforts. The Atrius quality teams generated monthly rosters of patients in need of services. Clinical teams worked from these lists, reaching out to patients whose diabetes or cardiovascular disease, for example, was not under control. Having both sets of data proved essential to the Atrius improvement efforts.

As the work progressed during the first year of the contract (2009), Lopez and Koplan worked to help clinicians identify and implement best practices. Part of that involved communicating clearly to the Atrius frontline staff what exactly the new contract entailed. In her presentations, Koplan emphasized that the "old way" was just a few metrics with minimal improvement expected and relatively few dollars at risk, whereas the "new way" was "thirty-plus ambulatory metrics across specialties, age groups, [and] service lines," where the goal was to "shoot for the moon." The progression, she said, would have to go from "good practice to best practice," and "standard work/evidence-based guidelines" would be essential elements as would "transparency—across [the] organization; by site; by individual docs."

The Atrius leadership was enthusiastic about the AQC from the start. "From our perspective at an organizational level," says Koplan, "the AQC was a good model for where we wanted to go—global payment, adjusted health risk status accompanied by transparent quality metrics across the board. We believed this was a good model for us and the right direction . . . [for] health care payment in the future."

Harvard Vanguard—the largest group practice within Atrius—had invested time and energy in the early part of the decade adopting aspects of the chronic care model developed by Dr. Edward H. Wagner at Group Health in Seattle. Wagner's approach relies on evidence-based care and clinical teamwork to treat patients with chronic conditions. (This was also the model adapted by HealthPartners and CareOregon in redesigning primary care.) Harvard Vanguard had also initiated team-based efforts with motivational interviewing and techniques for dealing with behavioral issues and had achieved some success with chronically ill patients. But the AQC required a much broader and more intensive effort. "We had to improve our understanding of those techniques and list them as a toolbox, as what you need to have in place to do this well," says Lopez. "Everybody wants to improve performance, but how exactly do you do it? It required crystallizing these approaches into easily explainable and generically adaptable approaches, which we did and shared with all the practices."

## Learning Together: The Quality Improvement Council

In 2009, Kate Koplan and Rick Lopez conceived what they called the Quality Improvement Council, which would prove to be a powerful catalyst for improvement. The idea was simple: every month, Koplan and the internal medicine leaders would select a single metric—LDL cholesterol control for people with diabetes, for example—then they would convene a meeting with the clinical leaders and their administrative partners from each of the twenty-one Atrius sites. The council included the chiefs of internal medicine and nursing and the administrative leaders of the groups that, at that time, made up the Atrius Health system. The monthly meetings followed a simple template. Koplan would kick things off with an explanation of the particular metric that was the focus of that session and that would be followed by presentations from high and low performers and then a robust discussion.

A meeting focusing on the AQC hypertension metric was typical of the Quality Improvement Council's work. Prior to the session the top two and the bottom two performers on this metric were asked to prepare a brief presentation about their site's work in this area. The point of the sessions was to identify themes that could help everybody improve, but particularly the lower performers. The meetings are "absolutely not punitive, not judgmental," says Koplan. The whole idea is to support a culture of improvement, to share improvement ideas and techniques, and to help lower performers identify and overcome barriers.

Koplan started the meeting with an overview of the metric, reminding the teams that hypertension "is the most common primary care diagnosis for adults in America" and that "effective treatment of hypertension has been associated with reductions in stroke incidence by 35 to 40 percent, heart attacks by 20 to 25 percent, and heart failure by more than 50 percent." She noted that performance on the AQC blood pressure metric had declined slightly in recent months and remained just below the goal for 2011. She discussed a variety of points that she suggested might be helpful to groups working to improve patients' blood pressure control. "Clinician awareness of and engagement with blood pressure goals" was central to the effort.

After Koplan spoke, representatives of the two lowest-performing sites made brief presentations followed by representatives of the two highest-performing sites. The physician representing the first low-performing site said she was disappointed that their numbers had declined and that they weren't yet exactly sure why. One possible explanation was that medical assistants were in some cases rounding up their numbers. The target was equal to or less than 139 over 89—which some medical assistants routinely rounded up to 140 over 90, which was too high. Koplan thought better communication with the medical assistants, and the clinicians, about the actual goal could help to make sure they understood it and recorded it precisely.

The representative from the second low-performing group said that they had a large number of DNKs (patients who "did not keep" their appointments) and they needed to identify a process for reducing the DNK rate. One possibility was to make live phone calls to patients with upcoming appointments as opposed to recorded calls.

What interested Koplan in both these cases was that lack of physician engagement in the work was not a factor in either case. "Two years ago they would have said, 'we are low because we haven't started yet,' but that doesn't happen anymore," she says. "It's never that they are not paying attention to the measure."

When the nurse leader from the first high-performing group went through her presentation, she said that things had gone well because clinicians were really engaged "and they worked hard to close the loop with follow-up. They had very engaged nurse-practitioners and medical assistants." She said, "We're just into this thing, we are just all over it." The representative from the second high performer said that this group, which was quite small, had no stringent system but that the entire team, led by the physicians, was engaged in the work and was aggressive about blood pressure management. The medical assistants were aware of the work and when they spotted a high blood pressure level they circled it so it was one of the first things the physician saw at the start of an appointment.

At the end of the sixty-minute Quality Improvement Council session, it was clear that doctors needed to be more aggressive about managing blood pressure medications for patients who were "just out of control." Koplan conveyed the message that a good deal of room remained for improvement in hypertension and that it remained high on the priority list.

"If everyone leaves with one or two ideas about how to do something new or buff up something, we have achieved our goal," says Koplan. And as she visits Atrius clinical sites, she invariably sees evidence of best practices learned from these meetings being spread.

## Targeting Practice Pattern Variation

These council meetings and other reviews of the data revealed the greatest challenge to improvement: widespread variation among the groups on their performance levels. Although some clinics would score at an exceptional level on a particular measure, other clinics might score 40 percent below that.

Variation meant uneven care under any contract, but variation also meant that Atrius was not doing everything possible to maximize its improvement scores under the AQC. Thus Lopez and other Atrius leaders dug into the variation issue with an effort to develop standardized clinical guidelines for physicians. "Why are some doctors ordering certain tests or procedures when the medical literature doesn't justify it?" asks Lopez. "There is *huge* variation there. A lot of doctors do things because that's the way they learned it and they don't know that the evidence shows that a different way is better and more efficient. So we have to analyze data with the clinical groups and have them all agree, on their own volition, what good care is based on the literature."

Lopez says that Atrius has done little about variation in the past but that is changing: "We're now beginning an intensive effort to look at practice pattern variation . . . and we can see that there is an opportunity to save millions of dollars if we could reduce some of the practice variation not based on evidence."

Perhaps the only value provided by this variation was that the achievement level reached by the best performer was the marker Lopez, Koplan, and their colleagues used to set goals for all of Atrius Health. They would identify the highest-performing site on any given metric—add a percentage point or two to that, and set it as the goal for the twenty-one clinical sites. "It resonates with clinical groups to say, 'We're not picking these targets out of the air. This site has achieved this so there is no reason why we can't all achieve it,'" says Lopez.

Often variation resulted from how intensively a site focused on a particular metric or how well standardized the supportive workflows were. Those who worked in a focused, consistent manner on a diabetes measure, for example, tended to perform well. Such *gap analysis* effectively identified specific areas for improvement, and Koplan would respond with very specific suggestions for how to improve.

Koplan and her senior project manager, Betsy Keener, would visit clinics and talk with doctors, nurses, medical assistants, and other staff, asking questions such as these: Do you use the rosters to do phone outreach to patients who need tests? Do you have a process by which nurses can manage certain populations in terms of blood pressure or cholesterol control? Do you meet in teams to review the rosters and come up with action steps for each patient? Do the medical assistants have a role in supporting clinicians in getting the needed tests done?

The goal, wherever appropriate, was to establish the standard work that would result in improvements in the top-tier metrics. Koplan and Keener worked to create a toolkit that was essentially a set of standards for managing the clinical process around top-tier conditions. In addition, Dr. Les Schwab, chief medical officer of Harvard Vanguard, led a major internal effort to create comprehensive clinical standard guidelines for diabetes management.

"We are now beginning to do more work at looking at other conditions where there is great variation in clinical practice, such as ordering lab tests for routine physicals, ordering of cardiac testing, the use of MRIs in the management of back pain, and the frequency of screening colonoscopies," says Lopez.

## Making a Breakthrough in Population Management

Even before the AQC was in high gear, all of the Atrius Health sites were working to find particular ways of improving. A clinical site in the city of Somerville, a short distance from both Cambridge and Boston, found it had a great deal of room for improvement in a number of areas. The site leaders thought they should more aggressively reach out to patients needing tests and screenings. Toward that end they hired some energetic college students on a per diem basis and trained them as "population managers" whose job was to reach out to patients and ask them to come in for needed tests. Results improved significantly. In 2008, the Somerville site had 10 percent of its diabetic patients with a cholesterol LDL <100 (the target). Just eighteen months later more than 50 percent of the patients had achieved that level, and the average LDL score improved for the patients of all six doctors at the Somerville site.

Koplan studied this work and found there was no other initiative in Somerville at the time that could have caused such an improvement. With such impressive results the other Atrius sites followed Somerville's lead in hiring population managers, and all experienced significant gains.

For years Harvard Vanguard had sought to fill this population management role by assigning it to existing staff. It would assign a nurse or medical assistant to do this work, but invariably that person would be drawn into more immediate work. "What always happened," says Koplan, "was that population management is not urgent, in-your-face, I-have-a-need-today, so people would always get drawn into dealing with the patient in front of them or the patient on the phone and the population management work would never get done." With the new system the necessary population management work was properly staffed and therefore could be routinely accomplished.

## Making Efficient Referrals

As we saw earlier in the chapter, an essential element to succeeding under the AQC is making sure that patients who need specialty care or hospitalization get it in a location that offers both high quality and cost effectiveness. This aspect of the AQC is remaking the way Atrius Health and other provider groups work and, in the process, shifting the health care landscape in Boston. Ideally, when an Atrius patient needs specialty care, he or she will go to an Atrius specialist. This will mean the use of the same electronic medical record, good communication between primary care doctor and specialist, and controlled cost of care. The worst situation is when a patient chooses to go to one of the most expensive hospitals in Boston and then, in effect, disappears into that system. "With capitated contracts it is important for us to direct care to high-quality providers or services which are at a lower cost," says Lopez. "For drugs, this means an equivalent generic versus a brand name. For hospital services, we want to work with hospital partners where there is a reasonable cost and they return patients to your care."

This issue is an essential determinant of whether Atrius can succeed under the AQC. It is so important that Atrius is referring fewer of its patients to the highest cost academic centers in Boston and developing strong connections with a high quality but lower costs center. Although all provide superb care, the higher cost hospital is both paid higher hospital and professional rates and does not consistently return patients back to the referring clinician for care.

It is important to note that some of the most prestigious academic medical centers in Greater Boston have taken on the AQC: At the start of 2012, Partners HealthCare includes Massachusetts General and Brigham and Women's and nine other hospitals, as well as 1300 primary care physicians and approximately 6000 specialty physicians.

## Challenges to the AQC

Thus far the AQC has resulted in improved quality metrics and, in some cases, control over costs, and it has proven highly popular with physicians and hospital leaders. But there have been dissenters, led by persistent questioning over time from Paul Levy, former CEO of Beth Israel Deaconess Medical Center. On his blog for March 17, 2011, *Running a Hospital* (retitled *Not Running a Hospital* after he stepped down as CEO), Levy cited a report from the Massachusetts inspector general that stated: "There is little doubt that fee-for-service reimbursements create incentives for providers to increase utilization of health care services, with obvious inflationary consequences. But moving to an ACO global payment system, if not done properly, also has the potential to inflate health care costs dramatically."

Levy saw this inflationary potential in the budgetary starting point of the AQC. "The capitated amounts are determined by starting with the previous year's experience of the population of lives covered by the specific AQC," he wrote. "That entire amount becomes the base year from which all future payments are derived. Therefore, the AQC embraces and adopts any excessive or wasteful payments in that base year, including all overutilization resulting from over a decade's worth of fee-for-service provider contracts. Implicitly, the premium increases of that decade, which overall were well in excess of 100 percent, are made a permanent part of our health care system's cost structure."

Levy further contends that those baseline budgets are inherently unequal due to the market power of some provider groups to gain greater reimbursements from Blue Cross. Levy also criticized a lack of transparency related to AQC contracts. He observed on his blog: "The IG's remarks are especially apt in that the first global contracts contained very good deals for those providers who signed on, as rewards for being early adopters. The big problem he identifies, as I have mentioned before, is the lack of transparency surrounding this issue. Absent an open presentation of rates and practice patterns, we will never know how effective this payment regime really is."

## Indications of Success So Far

Paul Levy's concerns, along with those of the state's inspector general, are serious and have to be taken as such. But even with certain flaws, the AQC has, at the very least, shown significant promise. And the study by Harvard Medical School researchers mentioned earlier indicates that the AQC "was associated with modestly lower medical spending and improved quality of care in its first year of use" (Song et al., 2011). A summary prepared by the Commonwealth Fund presents Song et al.'s key findings as follows:

- Health care spending increased for both ACQ and non-AQC enrollees. However, the quarterly increase was smaller for AQC enrollees—$15.51 less per enrollee.
- Medical procedures, imaging, and testing accounted for more than 80 percent of the savings. Care utilization rates were not significantly different, however, leading researchers to conclude that the savings derived largely from shifting outpatient care to providers that charged lower fees.
- The AQC was associated with improved performance on measures of the quality of adult chronic care and pediatric care, but not of adult preventive care. Quality improvements were likely due to a combination of substantial financial incentives and data support from Blue Cross Blue Shield.
- All AQC groups met 2009 budget targets and were eligible to share in the savings that accrued [Lorber, 2011].

It is important to recall that this study covered only the first year of the AQC, which is a five-year contract. Although it is possible that the quality gains will not be sustained, it appears far more likely that they will accelerate. In fact results from both Mount Auburn and Atrius Health after two years indicated significant quality improvement. Although the cost control side of the equation has been slower to take hold, both Mount Auburn and Atrius reported progress in that area as well in year two.

At Atrius, Lopez and his colleagues "feel very strongly in favor of global payment and value-based care." Done the right way nationally, Lopez believes the AQC approach has the potential to "bend the cost curve," and he notes, as an example, that through three consecutive quarters covering the end of 2010 and first half of 2011, Harvard Vanguard has "seen a reduction in quarterly increases in commercial PMPM [per member per month] total medical expense."

Lopez believes there are other broad social benefits accruing from the AQC as well. He suggests that global capitation—with significant bonus payments for quality—could well result in an overall increase in compensation for primary care doctors, thus improving their job satisfaction and potentially attracting more medical students into primary care. And he believes that the team-based primary care that the AQC fosters—necessitates, really—can also improve the quality of life for primary care doctors.

Moreover, Kate Koplan sees the work Atrius Health is doing with the AQC as well aligned with the Triple Aim. When it comes to population health, she notes that "all of the effectiveness measures in the AQC, plus at least twenty more (HEDIS and otherwise)" are published internally at least quarterly as part of the comprehensive quality dashboard at Atrius. She notes that there are eight patient experience measurements in the AQC and that Atrius also examines "the MHQP [Massachusetts Health Quality Partners] patient experience survey annually and the Press Ganey patient experience scores on an ongoing basis." Finally, in the area of efficiency, Koplan says that Atrius is working on "a broad array of initiatives—generics versus brand name drugs, advanced imaging metrics, et cetera. We are definitely actively working on creating more thorough Triple Aim reports. This is a big push moving forward."

## Keys to Doing This Work

A number of the individuals working with the groups discussed in this chapter have summarized the essential issues and ingredients to consider when adopting a contracting model similar to the Alternative Quality Contract.

*Steven J. Fox (Blue Cross Blue Shield of Massachusetts): Keys to AQC Success*

- **Widely accepted measures.** The measures are nationally accepted as clinically appropriate, so there is wide support for improving performance on these indicators.
- **Worthwhile rewards.** Real dollars are at stake for improvement.
- **A range of targets.** For each measure, there is a range of performance targets representing a continuum from good care to outstanding care, so the model rewards both performance and performance improvement.

- **Frequent performance reports.** Data are made available monthly, enabling the organizations to track progress and take action to manage their patient population.
- **Leadership support.** The groups have strong support from their leadership to implement new systems and act on the data [adapted from Fox, 2011, p. 24].

*Rick Lopez and Kate Koplan (Atrius Health): Keys to Success in a Provider Organization*

- **Availability of data.** Information is key. You need data to be able to identify opportunities for improvement and to measure the success of interventions. Use of data must be transparent for everyone to benefit from it.
- **Staff engagement.** Engagement of clinicians in the work—and their clinical teams—is critical to success.
- **Trusted leaders.** Credible physician leadership is a major factor in engaging clinicians and providing the right direction.
- **Highly effective teams.** Team efforts are crucial—everyone needs to be working "at the top of their license" and work distributed in standard ways to ensure that happens.
- **Standardization.** Reduction in practice variation is one of the most important factors in improving quality and reducing cost. This requires not only guidelines and the use of evidence-based medicine, but also the implementation of processes that reliably produce the outcome one is aspiring to achieve.
- **Strong care management.** Finally, care management of high-risk patients, end-of-life patients, patients in transitions of care, and chronic illness patients to ensure coordination and optimization of care is critical in providing better quality and reducing the cost of care for these most expensive patients.

*Rob Janett (MACIPA): Keys to Success for Leaders of Physician Organizations*

- **Willingness to change the culture.** Focus on physician engagement and culture change in the ACO environment.
- **Consistency.** Offer persistent steady physician leadership.
- **Clarity of purpose.** Set the example.

- **Ongoing clinical experience.** Although there are pressures to do the contrary, it is good to stay active in clinical practice:

   Maintains your credibility as a patient-focused clinician in the eyes of other physicians
   Helps maintain empathy with the challenges of clinical practice.

- **Involvement of others.** Early on in the program, bring physicians into the process.
- **A quality mindset.** Focus on quality improvement. Efficiency will follow.
- **An emphasis on accurate information.** Use valid and reliable data.
- **An emphasis on skills.** Educate first. Then talk about incentives.
- **Rewards for what works.** Positive incentives work better than negative incentives (incentives need to be substantial enough to capture the attention of the doctor).
- **A foundation for the work.** Begin the program only after there is a strong relationship between hospital and physicians.

### Barbara Spivak (MACIPA): Keys to AQC Success

- **Knowledge of where to improve.** Data that point to areas of improvement on the efficiency side.
- **Identification of high-risk patients.** Data that focus the care on high-risk patients.
- **Information that leads to action.** Data that are actionable for the physicians (names of patients that need screening; suggestions about how to improve blood pressure, sugar, and cholesterol, and so forth).
- **An ability to guide clinicians.** Physician leadership.

# 5

# Bellin Health

## *Improving Population Health with the Right Care at the Right Place and the Right Cost*

Bellin Health in Green Bay, Wisconsin, measurably improved the health scores of its employees by 10 percent while reducing the cost of its employee health coverage by 15 percent over an eight-year period, saving over $13 million. Applying the lessons of population health management learned from working with its own employees, Bellin then spread population management to hundreds of companies in Wisconsin and Michigan.

Bellin is an integrated health care delivery system that includes Bellin Medical Group with ninety-three primary care physicians and Bellin Hospital, a 167-bed acute care facility. Bellin has worked with the employees of 2,500 companies—and is on-site at seventy-four locations—in an effort to improve employee health and control costs. Bellin has been singularly successful on both scores. Overall in the companies where it has worked, Bellin has completed more than 65,000 health risk appraisals (HRAs) and improved employees' aggregate average scores from 71.4 to 75.2 on a 100-point scale, while reducing the level of high-risk scores—0 to 50 points—from 16.3 percent to 10.6 percent.

**Table 5.1. Results for Nine Employers Using Bellin Services**

| Company | 2009 Actual | 2009 Mercer Average | Difference |
|---|---|---|---|
| Company 1 | $5,800 | $8,945 | ($3,145) |
| Company 2 | $8,379 | $8,945 | ($566) |
| Company 3 | $7,805 | $8,945 | ($1,140) |
| Company 4 | $8,051 | $8,945 | ($894) |
| Company 5 | $8,011 | $8,945 | ($934) |
| Company 6 | $5,228 | $8,945 | ($3,717) |
| Company 7 | $6,183 | $8,945 | ($2,762) |
| Company 8 | $6,141 | $8,945 | ($2,804) |
| Company 9 | $6,363 | $8,945 | ($2,582) |

*Note:* Average cost is based on Mercer total employer health spend per employee plan. It is the average cost across the employee base that includes family members.

A 2009 Bellin survey of nine companies using the full Bellin menu of on-site services indicated that average health care costs for these firms were 21 percent below the national average (see Table 5.1). And Bellin has helped to control the cost of care for those companies, where costs run 10 to 20 percent below the Mercer average cost per employee. If the Bellin model were to be adopted on the national level, projections indicate that employers could save an estimated $63 billion.

## A New Path Forward

In 2000, Bellin Health faced a competitive situation that posed a deeply serious threat to the organization's viability. CEO George Kerwin, a forty-year Bellin veteran, took a hard look at the health care landscape and realized a new path forward was needed. "We realized we would have to make significant changes," says Kerwin. "We realized that overnight we could lose 25 percent of our business."

Kerwin stepped back and took inventory, placing all of Bellin's expenses under the microscope. He cut back in a number of areas, and as painful as it was, he was forced to trim some positions and services. Bellin Health continued, however, to provide significant care to needy patients throughout the community, with very limited reimbursement. But what really struck Kerwin was the news from his chief financial officer (CFO) that the projected cost to cover his own employees' health care in 2002 would rise by 30 percent, or about $3 million. These were truly disturbing numbers— dollar amounts that, over the long run, could not be sustained. "Our health benefit cost at the time was in the area of $10 million, which was a significant number for us and we realized we didn't really know how we were spending it," says Kerwin. "We didn't really know much about the costs that we were incurring. We realized that we didn't know anything other than we wrote the check every month for the health benefit. There was just no way we could afford to pay these rates for our own employees."

Kerwin and his leadership team examined the health plan design and studied the cost drivers. They found that their employees were not nearly as healthy as they could be, and that a fairly small percentage of employees consumed a high percentage of the overall health benefit. "We realized we needed to get better information about the way that we were spending the dollars," he says, "and we also realized that people using the health benefit needed to be more invested in the benefit, be more invested in their own health." At the same time the Bellin CFO conveyed the bad news about the projected premium increase, he also sent along a newspaper clipping about an Indiana hospital that had started a program where personal health nurses worked with employees to improve their health and control costs.

Kerwin pulled together a meeting that included representatives from the human resource department and from the department that supervised business accounts and a broker from the insurance plan covering Bellin Health's employees. This team realized that one of the problems Bellin faced was a lack of awareness among its employees about the impact of their health care spending habits on the company. Like most health care consumers in the United States, Bellin employees had little awareness of the impact their health—or lack of it—had on Bellin's finances, and little to no awareness of the direct impact health care costs had on the economic viability of the organization for which they worked. Kerwin wanted to change that. He needed Bellin's community of workers to understand that their health, and how they used health care services, had a direct impact on the company's financial well-being.

The first step toward awareness was asking employees to take a health risk appraisal, with the promise that those who did so would not have their health insurance premiums rise the following year. At the same time, Bellin increased the health insurance deductible somewhat but also offered a $20 per month premium discount for those completing an HRA. Kerwin and other senior leaders made an aggressive effort to speak to the employees in small-group settings and to convey to them the seriousness of the competitive situation and the importance of completing the HRAs. More than 90 percent of the employees completed the appraisals, which included a questionnaire but made use mostly of objective metrics such as body mass index, blood pressure, results of blood work, and similar indicators.

## The Keys to Employee Engagement

Once Bellin had a rich store of HRA data, says Kerwin, the next step was to get employees engaged in improving their health. An employee scoring below 60 on the HRA had to engage with a nurse who could function as a health coach or a primary care physician to create an improvement plan in order to remain eligible for a premium discount. "We were trying to get them engaged in their own health," says Randy Van Straten, vice president for Business Health Solutions at Bellin.

As the program progressed, Bellin took it to a third step, which was focused on accountability. Kerwin and his team tiered the premium costs in relation to employees' HRA scores, and these incentives were dramatic, with Bellin offering a premium discount of $750 for employees scoring 86+ on the HRA and a $250 discount for employees scoring 71 to 85. In addition, Bellin began to fund employee *health reimbursement accounts*— money employees can put toward co-pays or premium costs—for employees who had received 100 percent of the primary care and screenings appropriate for the employee's age and gender.

The premium incentive that was initiated to motivate employees and spouses to improve their scores was based on an analysis comparing health spending to HRA score. Health care services for a worker scoring near the top of the HRA scale cost $3,000 a year whereas care for someone at the lower end of the HRA scale costs double that. In 2006, for example, Bellin employees and their families scoring 86 or above on the HRA cost $3,286 whereas those scoring under 50 points cost $6,322. Three years later the top bracket cost $2,949 versus $6,236 for those scoring under 50.

The fourth and final step built upon the first three to try to create a culture of health within the organization. Reaching this level, the Bellin leaders thought, could be transformative. It could fundamentally alter how employees viewed not only their health benefit and its cost individually and collectively but also the way they viewed their own health. Kerwin wanted employees to be able to justly say that they were healthier because they worked in this new culture; because they worked at Bellin. But to get there, Bellin had to significantly improve its employees' engagement with primary care physicians. Too often Bellin employees were seeing specialists when it was unnecessary to do so, and they were receiving far less preventive and wellness care than they needed. The financial incentive here—as much as $1,000 per year—required employees and their spouses to be up to date on all age- and gender-specific tests and screenings.

In terms of timing, the organization's need to change and the employees' emerging desire to get healthier met at an ideal midpoint. In that first year 200 Bellin employees retook their HRAs after just ninety days and it turned out that their scores had improved by an average of nearly 10 points in that short period of time. It became clear that anyone fully engaged could make great progress quickly.

Although there was some grumbling among employees who felt the new approach was invasive, the much broader response was positive. Kerwin says there was "an overwhelming voice from people who said, 'you saved me from a disease I didn't know I had. You gave me the motivation to lower my cholesterol, lose weight, stop smoking. You really did all those things. During the health risk appraisal my spouse had something abnormal and it turned into an early chronic disease that we are managing much better.'"

A senior player on Kerwin's team was thirty-one-year Bellin veteran Pete Knox, vice president for regional clinical sales and services. Knox was responsible for work outside the hospital—the medical group, physician practices, employer strategies, population health strategies, the physician hospital organization, and the clinically integrated network. "And the question of course," says Knox, "is if people were receiving the preventative services for their age and gender, could we have caught things earlier and not had things lead up to these large claims?"

Within just two years, Bellin reduced the cost of its health coverage for employees by 33 percent, without resorting to any sort of rationing or broad benefit cuts. In eight years time, Bellin saved an estimated $13 million while simultaneously improving the measurable health scores of its workers—all of this while national trends for both cost and health were headed in the opposite direction.

Kerwin, Knox, and the rest of the team learned important lessons from those early experiences. They came to understand that there were three categories of people within their overall employee population: the high-risk, high-cost employees on one end of the spectrum, a middle group with average costs and risks, and the very healthy, low-cost employees on the other end. It was important to keep the well workers well and to target the high-cost employees, and Bellin aggressively did both. The crucial role of primary care was again illustrated by the fact that 75 percent of the employees with very large insurance claims had no preventive intervention for two years prior to that claim.

Making progress with the high-risk group is essential of course, but the Bellin experience suggests that "the real sweet spot over the long term," as Knox describes it, "is trying to impact that middle group and keep them out of the high-risk category and hopefully move them up the ladder to the well category."

The Bellin team learned as well that there were several key drivers for success: leadership by senior management, engagement among employees, adequate resources for the entire program but especially for coaching and managing the high-risk patients, and not least, beginning to create a culture of health.

## Taking the Bellin Method to Other Companies

Bellin Health's leaders were onto something.

In the first decade of the twenty-first century, a provider organization with a demonstrated ability to improve quality and reduce cost was a rare species. And this realization among Kerwin and his colleagues that Bellin was on to something special came as competition was bearing down on them and Bellin was working feverishly to improve its financial health.

It was at this juncture that Kerwin, Knox, and Van Straten discussed whether their ability to improve health and control cost within their own employee population might be more broadly applied. It was obvious to them that companies throughout Wisconsin and the nation were struggling mightily with their costs of health care, and Bellin's leaders decided that offering these companies the opportunity to hire someone with the ability to come in and stop the financial bleeding held enormous promise. Thus was born a new product line at Bellin Health called Business Health Solutions. The idea could not have been simpler: Bellin teams would go out to other companies and propose to do for them precisely what they had done for their own employees. "We had the numbers," says Pete Knox. "When we went to a company back then it was basically, 'look what we did. We took about 33 percent of the cost off of our books for our health benefit by restructuring our plan, creating health awareness through health risk appraisals, and hiring people to help those who were at risk get better health.'"

What made the Bellin story even more impressive was that traditionally, health care provider organizations tended to have higher overall spending on care for their employees than companies in other industries. Perhaps this was due to a greater awareness of health-related issues. Whatever the cause, the cost was traditionally higher and thus Bellin's ability to cut the cost of paying for its own employees' health care from above to below average attracted some attention.

Bellin had the numbers on the quality improvement side as well—these were the numbers that made the financial side work. In 2002, the overall HRA score among Bellin's employees was 70.3 (again, that is on a 100-point scale), below the national average of 73.1. Just two years later the overall Bellin score had moved up to 72.6 compared to the then national rate of 70.8. (And in 2011, Bellin's score was 77.2 compared to 70.6 nationally.) Perhaps just as significant as those numbers was the improvement among employees with the lowest HRA scores. In 2002, 17 percent of Bellin employees had scored in the 0 to 50 range on the HRA.

By 2010, that had dropped to just 7 percent. (At no time did Bellin target lower-scoring employees for layoffs.)

The Bellin approach was built on a "fundamental belief that having a medical home primary care relationship is critical to the long-term success for a population," says Knox. "We realize that there are a lot of determinants of health that we don't directly influence and need to be working with others to impact. The key resource we bring to the table is primary care and the primary care team."

Bellin had an existing business unit that provided on-site occupational health services to employers and it built the new Business Health Solutions division on that platform. One significant advantage the business had at the start was that during the time the business unit had worked on improvement at Bellin, that unit had treated Bellin as a client, as a separate entity. This meant that it had the systems in place to deal with outside companies in almost exactly the same way its staff had performed their work with Bellin employees for several years.

However, because Bellin no longer has a health plan as part of its company and because it does not hold an insurance license, it is not permitted to engage in risk contracting. This raised a question about the finances of Business Health Solutions. Although the ideal contract for its work with employers might have been something along the lines of the Alternative Quality Contract discussed in Chapter Four—a contract where the organization would be rewarded financially for providing measurably better care—that is not an option available to Bellin. Thus all its work to date in Business Health Solutions has been under a kind of fee-for-service arrangement, though not the traditional fee-for-service in which providers are paid for volume. Bellin is paid by employers for the time of doctors, nurses, and physical therapists. "When we provide a nurse, they pay us for the nurse," says Knox. "They pay us for the provider. It's not the widget fee-for-service."

Initially, Bellin offered these services at cost (or even at a bit of a loss), confident that engagement with the companies would drive volume in the rest of their business—through primary and specialty care as well as the hospital. And that has proven true.

Kerwin, Knox, and Van Straten began visiting employers and telling the Bellin story. Their pitch included the notion that providing on-site health care cuts down on lost work time and thus increases productivity. When workers can be seen by care providers at the job site, it improves both their health and the company's bottom line.

## Drawing on Deep Community Roots

There was another important factor in those early days when Kerwin, Knox, and Van Straten—as well as a sales team—were out meeting with companies and making their pitch. It was an element that Bellin Health's major competitors could not match. Bellin had deep, sturdy roots in the Green Bay community. Kerwin, Knox, and Van Straten were all Green Bay natives who had spent virtually their entire professional careers at Bellin. They have been there forty, thirty-one, and twenty-seven years respectively. Van Straten had started working at Bellin part time at age eighteen in 1981 to help pay for college! The three men knew the leaders of just about every major company—and many smaller companies—in the area. "We felt if we could get a handle on the increasing costs of the benefit," says Knox, "and could control that ourselves, that with our relationships in the community we could take that out into the community and help other organizations do the same thing and it could end up being a competitive advantage."

That is not to say it was easy to sell companies on the concept. Many employers, in fact, had invested money in wellness programs during the 1990s with little if any benefit to their employees' health or to the company's bottom line. But there was a difference between a wellness vendor making a standard pitch and the Bellin executive team coming in and sitting down to talk with people they knew—neighbors and even friends in some cases. Knox jokes that during the early rounds of visits to employers, "some of them probably thought maybe we were building a new hospital wing and were going to ask for money."

Their pitch was solid. They had their own results to show of course. And they also had the infrastructure in place to support a serious wellness management program. "We had primary care, we had fitness centers, we had all the linkages together, and we actually brought [the program into] a health care system and then also worked with [a client company's] insurance broker to hardwire the plan into the benefit design," says Knox. "This approach brings the insurer, the employer population, and the health care system all working together." Another reason brokers were key was the close and trusted relationships many of them have with the employers they serve.

Early on, the Business Health Solutions division focused on one metric: the total amount a company spends on health care for its employees. This was unique, at least in this market. Nobody else was coming to these companies and saying that their program could reduce the total outlay (or *spend*)—not slow the rate of growth but actually reduce the total amount of money the company was spending on health care. "A metric of total spend was music to the ears of the benefits manager because no one had ever talked about that before," says Kerwin. Typically in the past, he says, providers complained about health plans and their excessive and intrusive administrative burdens while health plans complained about the variation and lack of cost controls among providers.

Kerwin was convinced that the total spend would tell the true story of what was happening with the health of an employee population. He believed that if Bellin's people could get into some companies and show what they could do, that significant breakthroughs were within their grasp. "Total spend was an indicator of health," says Kerwin. "If the health benefit was brought under control that was an indicator of health, so having that one metric was very unique and we *knew* we could produce for them."

Bellin's leaders also knew the potential market was very large because in the Greater Green Bay market more than 350,000 people—more than half of the total population—received their health coverage from an employer. Moreover the new product was flexible. The precise services Bellin provided depended entirely on customer needs. "Some companies chose to just work on health plan design," says Kerwin, "some chose to invest in health risk appraisals, some chose to do health risk appraisals and feedback and have on-site providers."

The Business Health Solutions mantra, says Van Straten, who runs the division, is "listen, design, deliver. We go out and listen to what the customer needs and design a solution *for them*, and then deliver it with accountability."

## A Model That Works for Large Employers ...

Among the first companies Bellin worked with on population health was American Foods Group, a large meat-packing firm located in Green Bay. Meat packing can be a physically demanding occupation, says Van Straten. "There are cuts and strains and various injuries and in that account they wanted to work on their injury claims." Some research into records including claims data revealed the opportunity for prevention strategies and treatment of injuries and accidents. Bellin put an occupational medicine physician on-site at the plant not only to deal with ongoing issues but also to try to build preventive measures into the work process. Bellin also placed a physical therapist on-site to do some treatment and to work on preventive ergonomics.

Van Straten says Bellin worked to configure its delivery of services to meet the employer's needs. A small yet telling example involves an initial health strategy that requires drawing blood to measure cholesterol levels among meat-packing plant workers. Pulling employees off the plant floor for any length of time could slow the production line, so rather than a traditional blood draw to test for cholesterol, the Bellin team used very quick finger sticks. "We had to work around the production lines and respect their efficiency," Van Straten says.

Over time, Bellin was able to educate many American Foods Group employees in pursuing better health through more diligent use of prevention and screenings and lifestyle changes that addressed smoking, nutrition, and weight. Another critical element was improving how and where the workers accessed the health care system. Unnecessary use of clinic visits and the emergency department declined once services were brought on-site, and this also helped to lower overall costs.

## ... and for Smaller Ones

A key decision early on was that Bellin would work with companies of just about any size. Kerwin and his team recognized that small and medium-sized companies were just as burdened by health costs as large companies and needed just as much help.

Although many organizations that work in this area feel that a very large number of employees is required to do this work, Bellin demonstrated an ability to configure a solution to each specific population set.

In those early days, Bellin also worked closely with HC Miller, a Green Bay supplier of office products such as binders and folders. The folks at HC Miller told Van Straten that they wanted to focus on improving the general health of their employees by having a primary care provider on-site.

Bellin's first step was to have the employees fill out a health risk appraisal and then to use the results to advise employees on what they might do to improve their overall health. A nurse was assigned to work at the HC Miller site two days a week, meeting with workers individually to coach and train them on improvement and wellness techniques. Anyone scoring under 60 on a health risk appraisal was assigned to a health coach, and the coach and a primary care physician, in collaboration with the employee, would establish an improvement program.

"Then," reports Van Straten, "the HC Miller folks said to us, 'Well, you guys are helping us with our health benefit; we are also having problems with our workers' comp or work-related injuries. Can you get a physical therapist in here to be on-site on a regular basis not just to treat our injured folks but to look ergonomically at our production systems and create a prevention program along with early intervention?' And we did. And that is a key part—early intervention for prevention." The program quickly expanded from there to include providers on-site at HC Miller to offer a range of services from writing prescriptions to dealing with acute care for illness and injuries that could be handled on-site. This meant faster, more convenient treatment for workers and lower costs for the company.

"Bellin Health is a partner and has had a huge impact on our organization," says Lynn Peterson, former human resource director for HC Miller. "We've seen the results of working with Bellin the past three years in lowered health care costs for both health care and workers' compensation. We've had less downtime, higher productivity, and healthier employees. Our health has been elevated to another level with Bellin helping with this initiative."

Bellin's new product continued to be a replica of what Bellin had done with its own employees. The Business Health Solutions team packaged what had been done internally, replicating the way Bellin had communicated with employees and the sequence and scheduling of various elements. The team copied almost exactly the letters that had been written to Bellin's own employees about HRAs and various health prevention and wellness benefits. The Bellin team members also found that they continued to learn important lessons within their own system that they then applied to various other companies. "We had early success replicating our experience within other companies and we continued to use ourselves as a proving ground, kind of a research area of this whole initiative," says Knox.

Within the Business Health Solutions approach lies the answer to one of the most intractable problems faced by primary care physicians throughout the United States every day—how to get at between-visit care. These primary care doctors and their teams struggle to connect with patients in between visits to the clinic. They use e-mail and phone calls to try to maintain communication, but it is often a challenge to coordinate. The Bellin approach is a breakthrough because it transports primary care teams out of the clinic and places them where the patients are located. Rather than a patient having to travel to the care team for periodic visits, the care team travels to the patient and is routinely available.

## Committing to Listen, Design, and Deliver

An essential element in the early marketing of Business Health Solutions was the enthusiastic and vocal support of the CEO of American Foods Group. When he spoke about improved health among his workers and reduced cost, he had great credibility with the leaders of other companies.

The importance of the *listen, design, deliver* mantra is hard to overstate. When Bellin engaged in discussions with a large bank in Green Bay, the bank was interested in having acute care services on-site. But when Van Straten, his team, and the bank's HR department and brokers sat down to review claims data, they didn't see much of a need for acute care. What they *did* see, however, was a need for care of chronic conditions. "An acute clinic would not have addressed their needs with chronic diseases," says Van Straten. "We went back with a proposal for an on-site nurse to coach workers on chronic disease management, and it has worked very well. It's some of the best engagement I've seen with any customer."

The resources Bellin brings to bear in any given company have depended entirely on the company's particular needs. In general Bellin provides some level of primary care—ranging from on-site physicians to a nurse available by phone. Beyond that, the specific needs have defined whether there are additional specialty services. For example, a plant where blue-collar workers experience numerous musculoskeletal issues might require an on-site physical therapist.

In its first couple of years of offering the new services, Bellin had considerable success. In a dozen or more companies of varying size and in different kinds of businesses, it demonstrated an ability to control costs while improving the health of employees. At each company the Bellin team found management passionate about somehow getting control of employee health care costs but deeply uncertain about what to do. Often the team encountered frustrated company leaders feeling as though the health benefit was out of control and fearful about where costs were headed in the future. And uniformly the team found employers not only eager to reduce costs but also wanting to have a healthier employee base in order to maintain or increase productivity.

As Bellin got its new business up and running, Knox retained the services of an experienced researcher, who dug deep into medical literature to provide a summary of the best thinking concerning the essential drivers of behavioral change. This was a tough issue. It was exceedingly difficult for people who were overweight to lose weight; it was hard for people to alter unhealthy eating habits; it was an arduous uphill battle for people to quit smoking or cut back on alcohol use. But Knox wanted to know the very latest scientific thinking on what worked and what did not work in this area. "What were the drivers of success in behavior change?" he asked. "What could we do to support people more effectively?"

This research did not of course find any silver bullets. But it—as well as the Bellin team's practical experience—did show that consistency of effort is essential, as is goal setting and engagement between the patient and the coach. And working with people *before* they were ready to change was futile—but staying in touch with them so that programs were readily available once they were ready was crucial. Knox also learned that people with multiple behavioral issues are quite often ready to change in one area (losing weight, for example), but not in another (such as stopping smoking). "We learned that the motivation needed to be intrinsic rather than extrinsic," he says. Even if the change effort starts out as extrinsic, it must quickly shift over to being intrinsic to the individual or it will quickly fail.

As it did with its own employees, Bellin looks at each population it works with in three broad categories: low-risk, at-risk, and high-risk. The Bellin team recognized that the health and lifestyle issues of its own workers were quite similar to many other employee populations. With low-risk workers the goal is to help them maintain their good health with preventive screenings, wellness campaigns, and where necessary some health coaching. At the other end of the spectrum are the high-risk workers who typically are experiencing such serious maladies as diabetes, hypertension, obesity, or coronary artery disease. Most cigarette smokers tend to be in the high-risk category. When people in this category are ready to change, Bellin comes in full force with various programs and coaching.

As Bellin found with its own employees, the at-risk group is critically important. Bellin has worked to, first and foremost, help these people at least stay where they are and not slip into the high-risk category. This is essential for their health and for overall costs. And when progress is made here—using targeted interventions and screenings, stress management, coaching, and more—people can move into the low-risk category. When this happens, it is of course both a health and financial triumph.

## Understanding That One Size Does Not Fit All

The Fincantieri Marine Group is a shipbuilding company with facilities in Green Bay, Marinette, and Sturgeon Bay, Wisconsin. The facilities in Marinette and Sturgeon Bay, run by Fincantieri sister subsidiaries Marinette Marine Corporation and Bay Shipbuilding, respectively, reported that less than 11 percent of their workers were getting annual physicals and 80 percent of them did not have a primary care physician. Fincantieri Marine had a disease management program in place, but less than 1 percent of the workers participated. In addition, the numbers showed that workers and their families had very low immunization rates.

Not surprisingly, the facilities' health care costs were climbing at an unsustainable pace. From 2009 to 2010, for example, these costs climbed 44 percent. Sarah Novak, compensation and benefit manager at Marinette Marine Corporation/Bay Shipbuilding, solicited proposals from providers, looking for someone who could improve care quality and control costs among the employees. One provider made a very attractive proposal to pay for and install a trailer on-site to house primary care services. This company offered a series of services at low or no cost, with the apparent goal of using its work at Marinette Marine Corporation/Bay Shipbuilding as a template for expanding into the marketplace. Another provider made a somewhat similar offer. But when Novak met with its representatives, they told her there was no room for flexibility, that the template they had built would be in place and there would be "no tweaks."

Novak had made up her mind to go with the first provider and met with Bellin in 2010 only as an afterthought. But after talking with Van Straten and his team, she believed Bellin was the right choice. Bellin had by then been successful with this work in more than forty companies, and Novak says, "Randy and his team were open to ideas on how to make the clinics work and be successful. They understood that one size does not fit all."

Van Straten promised her that if she chose Bellin he would have the primary care trailer up and running within ninety days. Van Straten stressed that the program was a partnership; that he and his team would work with her to get the employees—and the bottom line—to a much better place. Van Straten made good on his ninety-day promise, and it quickly became clear that the convenience of the on-site services—coaching, counseling, blood work, and so forth—was a difference maker.

"A lot of credit goes to Sarah and her team," says Van Straten. "She was determined to get her employees and their families more engaged with their health. . . . Sarah's vision was to get health care close and convenient for the workers and their families and to remove barriers to care." For patients with chronic conditions, such as diabetes, cholesterol, and hypertension, testing was easily and quickly done on-site. And to encourage employees to stay on medication, the co-pay for diabetic medications was waived. "It made it so much more convenient to get lab work done on-site," Novak says. "Because I know that otherwise . . . [the employees] won't get the lab work done."

Novak did not have a large number of claims for health insurance payments to providers, but the ones she did have were generally very large, and many were related to heart and respiratory diseases. She worked with local providers in Sturgeon Bay and Marinette, seeking health care discounts for her workers and met with some success.

Although this program is still in the early stages of operations with its on-site clinics, hard dollar savings are already near $100,000. However, Novak says that does not represent the true total savings. She says that data are "already showing that potential very high cost catastrophic cases are being identified early and prevented because of removing the barriers of cost and convenience with the engagement of primary care. That is where the true savings are and what this strategy is about."

## Breakthrough

For all the success Business Health Solutions has had, the work is not easy and progress is often incremental. At some companies Bellin could not start by administering HRAs and gaining critical data because some union shops were wary of what employers might do with that information.

"The question with any employer is what pieces of the puzzle are you willing and able to put in place today?" says Knox.

> You want to put primary care on-site—that is a good start. You are not ready to do health risk appraisals. We think that is pretty important. We would like to try to work with you over time to get there, but we are not going to say no to you unless you are willing to buy our whole puzzle and all the pieces. Do we think and believe strongly that that is an important thing for you to do? Yes.

So what we do in almost every case is we will talk about the whole picture. Very few companies say, "Great, let's do it all tomorrow." So we will go in and say, "Where are you at today? Let's start working where you are at, where you are comfortable. Let's start there."

There are times where we have asked ourselves, should we walk away from business because a company is not willing in a sense to do what we think is necessary? We have not made that decision to walk away. We have made the decision "let's get in and establish a base and keep working with them over time to implement the rest of the model, demonstrate results, develop a relationship with whatever the case may be." There are organizations that have unions that just cannot go there today. So we say, "We will work with you if we start over here and try to work there." So that has been our approach.

Since it launched Business Health Solutions, Bellin has engaged with over 2,500 companies, ranging from self-employed truckers to a Georgia Pacific paper mill with three thousand employees. The business health solutions model is now in seventy-four sites where, depending upon the size of the company, Bellin may have simply a virtual clinical relationship to site, or a robust on-site presence including a physician, registered nurse, and physical therapist.

When Bellin goes into a company and establishes a full beachhead with a combination of a consumer-driven health plan, on-site services, employee HRAs, and incentives for participation, the results are health care costs 10 to 20 percent below the national average.

## The Essential Ingredients

It was clear by 2006 that Bellin's Business Health Solutions division was succeeding due to the integration of various elements. Until that time, Kerwin and his team had not defined precisely how they thought about the elements or how exactly they all fit together, but by 2006 they were thinking in a broad way about what the elements were and how they worked. After a series of internal discussions, Kerwin, Knox, and Van Straten came up with the term *total health model* to reflect their belief that an integrated set of services could provide precisely what the name implied.

Knox had led an internal effort at Bellin to conduct a fairly exhaustive literature search looking at what employers were doing to improve health and to reduce cost for their employee populations. That study, along with the Bellin leaders' own knowledge and experience, led them to identify the following five components of the total health model that they believed were essential to successful population health management at any organization.

## Leadership and Culture

In considering this first component, the fundamental question, in Knox's words, is whether the organization's leaders have "created a culture which is aligned with health and wellness." At Bellin, for example, Knox points out that "you could walk into our cafeteria four or five years ago and it would look very different than it does today." Instead of the wide variety of foods heavy on fat and calories that you would have found then, there is now a far more balanced offering. Any employee wishing to eat a healthy, satisfying meal now has many different choices. And the most egregious sorts of fatty, unhealthful foods have all but disappeared from the cafeteria offerings.

"In a sense [the question is] are we putting our money where our mouth is?" says Knox. "Are we willing to make changes in the environment, policies, and rules?" Are leaders at Bellin willing to demonstrate a commitment to health and wellness in their own lives, in their level of activity and exercise, in their lifestyle habits related to the use of tobacco and alcohol, in their nutritional choices? How "[we leaders] act and how we behave as a group, we believe, is fundamental to any long-term change."

## Health Knowledge

The second component of the model involves developing a deep understanding of the population and its members' health risks as well as the major drivers of cost. And populations can be very different. Knox points out, for example, that Bellin works with a foundry where the workers are male with an average age of forty-five and also with a bank where most of the employees are females in their twenties. The needs of each of these populations will be "quite different and that is going to drive different solutions," says Knox. To gather knowledge of a population's health, Bellin teams mine "anything and everything we can get our hands on" including claims data, health risk assessments, disability and workers' comp claims, and focus group interviews. They want to understand the population they are dealing with so they can find the most productive avenues to better health and also so they can identify areas where incentives can be aligned to promote the choices that will improve the health of the population.

## Health Advancement

This third component of the model involves an intensive focus on managing chronic conditions through a variety of means, including lifestyle and behavioral change. Says Knox: "In health advancement we are really trying to support the individual in making health decisions, and bringing the resources necessary to them to make changes in their lives or support them in those changes."

## Productivity Enhancement

The fourth component includes a variety of health and wellness services along with rehabilitation, including physical and occupational therapy. It also includes an ergonomic analysis of the workplace to ease the physical strains on workers and prevent injuries. Health and workplace productivity are inextricably linked. They are so intertwined, in fact, that working on improving health provides a direct benefit to improving workplace productivity as well as overall quality of life.

## Navigation Platform

The fifth and final component of the model is a navigation platform where the goal is to design a series of access points to care for patients, access points that make it easy for people to get the services they need—the right care in the right place at the right cost.

## Right Care, Right Place, Right Cost

If the business health solutions model is one of Bellin's greatest innovations, the other is its navigation platform. Getting patients to access care in the right setting, at the right time, and for the right price is one of the central challenges in health care in the United States. Throughout this country, substantial *unnecessary* costs arise when people access care in a location ill suited to their needs. In Bellin's model, the entry point for the navigation platform is a nurse call line. When Van Straten and his team go into a company they provide every employee with a card bearing a single phone number; that number will connect the employee, at any time of day or night, to an on-duty nurse. That nurse's job is to guide the person to exactly the right level of care for whatever ails him or her.

Every nurse answering the phone line is highly knowledgeable, with a keen understanding of the precise benefits provided by every company with which Bellin works. The nurse consults a computer screen and sees, for example, what the caller's co-pay, if any, is for a visit to FastCare (a Bellin primary care service described in the next section). By guiding patients to the right care setting, the nurse is both responding to each patient's needs by supplying a specific solution and serving the needs of the company by controlling costs. People do not suddenly decide to break old habits—such as going to the emergency department—right away. However, Bellin mounts a comprehensive communication effort in each company to make clear to employees that when they have a problem their first stop should be the nurse call line, and fairly quickly employees discover that the nurse triage system works well for them and their families.

This approach emerged from what Bellin had done for its own employees in arranging access to care (see Figure 5.1). "We designed this to say to employees that these are low-cost, very efficient ways for you to access care all the way up through primary care, into specialty care, the emergency department, and ultimately tertiary care," says Kerwin, "but you should start at the most inexpensive appropriate way of accessing."

## Figure 5.1. Health Care Navigation—Delivering Care

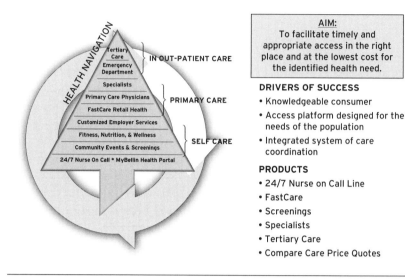

**AIM:**
To facilitate timely and appropriate access in the right place and at the lowest cost for the identified health need.

**DRIVERS OF SUCCESS**
- Knowledgeable consumer
- Access platform designed for the needs of the population
- Integrated system of care coordination

**PRODUCTS**
- 24/7 Nurse on Call Line
- FastCare
- Screenings
- Specialists
- Tertiary Care
- Compare Care Price Quotes

*Source:* Bellin Health.

## FastCare: Less Expensive Care

The Bellin team found that although the nurse telephone line they originated in 2005 worked well, there was an opportunity gap in access between the nurse line and primary care visits. They believed there was ample space between the phone service and primary care visits for a more easily accessed, retail-level clinic where a large majority of standard complaints could be handled quickly, effectively, and inexpensively. To fill this space and expand the primary care platform, Bellin created FastCare, primary care clinics staffed by nurse practitioners and physician assistants who can provide basic care for a wide variety of common ailments. FastCare clinics are set up next to existing pharmacies in retail spaces that are well known and easily accessible to patients. The clinics are open from 8:00 AM to 8:00 PM, 365 days a year.

Kerwin explains the team's thinking this way:

> [After talking to the on-duty nurse, people] would get an appointment with a primary care physician for the next morning,

come in to that appointment, get the diagnosis from the primary care physician, get the prescription, and then go to the pharmacy, get the prescription filled, and start . . . [their] child on that prescription regimen. We have thousands of people going through this and it is inefficient because it is not an emergency—it is something that could be easily diagnosed, they still have to go to the pharmacy, so we developed this thinking to take the care to the pharmacy, basically, in a retail setting, so you get more hours of coverage, the mom can go in and have everything done at one time—a much more efficient system.

Van Straten cites a Commonwealth Fund survey from 2007 indicating that two-thirds of Americans say they have difficulty getting care on nights, weekends, and holidays, and just 30 percent of Americans can get into see their doctor on the same day they call and ask for care (Schoen et al., 2011). A more recent Commonwealth Fund survey (2011), indicates that 55 percent of patients face difficulty in getting access to care after hours without going to the Emergency Department. When FastCare is available, however, "if you have the flu or a cold or your child wakes up and has an earache, you take them into this very efficient clinic that happens to be right next to a pharmacy," says Kerwin.

In Bellin's program some problems can be handled by the nurse on the call line, others by FastCare clinics. When something is more acute, the nurse is empowered to set up a primary care clinic appointment for the following day. All of this requires an aligned and complete primary care platform with open access to the medical home. "The navigation platform works best when companies align their health plan to support the navigation platform," says Van Straten. "For example, at Bellin, we waived the deductible and offered free FastCare services in our plan, and we saw a 64 percent decrease in ER visits for coded level 1 and 2 visits. That's a $52 visit versus a $600 visit."

Van Straten says there are some payers—notably Medicaid— that will pay for an emergency department (ED) visit but not for a FastCare visit. Thus a person who might well be taken care of efficiently, quickly, and inexpensively at a FastCare site would likely opt for the ED if the out-of-pocket difference was $52, the fee for a FastCare clinic visit. But Bellin revamped its own health plan so that any employee who goes to FastCare has the fee waived, and many companies for whom Bellin works on population health have followed suit. The value of getting patients to FastCare rather than the primary care clinic or the emergency department is worth vastly more than $52 to the companies. And in many companies, treatment at FastCare clinics is free when patients use them to stay on track for chronic care treatment or when they use FastCare as an alternative to the emergency department.

## A Link to Primary Care

FastCare clinics are sometimes used by physicians wanting to follow up with patients who have chronic conditions and need to have their cholesterol, blood pressure, or blood sugars checked, for example. It is quick and easy for patients and helps unclog primary care clinics. The Bellin team has discovered that FastCare settings are excellent for school physicals and also help reduce the volume at pediatric clinics.

All of these instances in which clinical work is funneled to FastCare are generally faster for patients and much less expensive for patients and employers. In addition, getting so many routine cases to the appropriate care setting means that primary care physicians are able to spend more time on higher-end, more challenging cases. Bellin data support this conclusion, showing conclusively that with the rising popularity and use of FastCare, there has been a meaningful decrease in the use of Bellin Hospital's emergency department. At the same time, says Knox, the data clearly show that "the acuity level in primary care has gone up," enabling physicians to spend more time on the more complex problems that they are trained to handle. "It has been significant in our primary care practices," says Knox. The data show that in primary care doctors see many fewer relatively simple, straightforward cases, such as earaches, sore throats, and the like. Meanwhile, says Knox, "We have seen a migration toward level 4s and 5s [that is, toward more intensive care] in our outpatient practice."

For the overall approach to work, says Knox, FastCare must be an extension of the primary care setting. "It is an acute care product being delivered somewhere else," he says. "The electronic medical record links back into the medical home, and the physician and the care team are still in control of that care." In addition, says Knox, the Bellin medical director reviews records on all FastCare visits and "I can tell you and he would tell you that we actually do a better job of following protocol in our FastCare clinics than we do anywhere else. It is a more basic need that is being met. Protocols are pretty well defined and pretty specific."

FastCare has grown to become the largest health system–based retail clinic brand in the United States, with fifty-seven clinics in fifteen states either open or under construction. These clinics are operated by thirty-three different health systems and see about seven thousand patients per clinic each year.

## QuadMed

Of course, Bellin is not the only organization providing high-quality workplace care. QuadMed in Sussex, Wisconsin (ninety-three miles from Green Bay) is one of the pioneers in employer-sponsored, worksite health care and a member in the IHI Triple Aim Collaborative. One of the more remarkable stories in modern American health care, QuadMed was started in 1990 by the owners of a large printing company, Quad/Graphics. The ownership was frustrated with the quality and cost of care for their employees and made the decision to bring that care in-house and provide it directly to employees in the workplace. The result was better care at a lower cost for Quad/Graphics' 28,000 employees and their families. Estimates are that QuadMed spends approximately 30 percent less to cover their employees than comparable companies in their state. The method is very similar to that used by Bellin— aggressive primary care on-site focused on wellness and prevention. The Quad/Graphics work was so successful that QuadMed was formed to provide on-site services to other companies.

### Pursuing the Triple Aim

In 2009, as they regularly do, the members of the Bellin leadership team had an in-depth strategy discussion. They had accomplished a great deal since those difficult days years earlier when they had struggled against an intense competitive threat. Since then, they had succeeded in building a robust primary care network and a full array of specialty care, and had greatly enhanced relationships with physicians. They had created and spread Business Health Solutions and FastCare, constructed a powerful navigation platform, and achieved financial stability.

The question in 2009, as Kerwin convened his senior team to discuss the future, was *what next?* What should they do to maximize the effectiveness of their organization's capabilities? "We began to look at a more aggressive, even more outwardly focused mission and strategy that addressed the health of the entire population," says Kerwin.

Knox recalls that the discussions "started with a blank sheet of paper" and a question: "Here's where we are and here's where the world is going—what do we want to pursue in the future?" It was clear in 2009, says Knox, that the future belonged to provider organizations able to manage population health effectively. Thus the Bellin leadership looked to the future and envisioned moving toward a much more robust community engagement, via primary care, to manage the health of the Greater Green Bay population. Their discussions led them to a new vision and mission statement. The current Bellin mission statement says:

> Bellin Health is a community-owned not-for-profit organization responsible for the physical and emotional health of people living in Northeast Wisconsin and the Upper Peninsula of Michigan.
>
> Directly, and in partnership with communities, employers, schools, and government officials, we guide individuals and families in their lifelong journey toward optimal health. We are committed to providing safe, reliable, cost-effective total health solutions with respect and compassion. Our innovative work will impact healthcare delivery in our region, as well as throughout the world.

Bellin's vision statement says: "The people in our region will be the healthiest in the nation."

Bellin Health would continue doing what it had been doing in a variety of areas. There would be no let up in anything that was working. But the organization would begin a journey toward population health management as never before, with the Triple Aim embedded in its mission.

When the original IHI Triple Aim program started in 2007, Bellin Health joined it, acting on the leaders' belief that Bellin's work for several years had been, without labeling it as such, Triple Aim focused. And certainly Business Health Solutions was an example of getting at an improved patient experience, better population health, and lower costs. To broaden the effort to the entire regional population of 600,000 was another matter, however, and until 2009, Bellin had not been in a position to take on such an ambitious goal. Knox talks about Bellin having had to "earn the right to innovate" by getting foundational elements in place, elements that would facilitate improving the patient experience (including quality of care), improving the health of the population, and lowering cost. "If you don't have a stable platform or production system your ability to take that and innovate off of it is minimized," he says. "So when we looked at primary care we looked at can you go out and sell our total health model if we have not standardized open access across the system."

Essential to the success of a health care model is a reliable production system, says Knox, and he defines this system as the resources, assets, processes, and knowledge required to design and produce a product or service. "If we weren't doing disease management efficiently in our core production system, our ability to take that out with any confidence and offer it in a different environment would be pretty minimal," he says. "So I think the concept behind production system design is [that] you have got a stable core production system. You are efficient with that. It allows you to extend and expand the boundaries of the production system, offer new features, innovate across it pretty quickly."

Unless the production system within Bellin is consistent and reliable, very little of what the leaders attempt to do will succeed, says Knox. "If we were in our old world and every clinic were doing things differently—if the chassis or platform was different in thirty-five separate clinics and we came along with a great idea that we thought would advance primary care and we tried to implement that in thirty-five sites that were doing things differently we would be managing thirty-five very distinct changes. The prospect of being successful with that is next to zero."

Participating in the IHI Triple Aim initiative gave Bellin three clear dimensions on which to focus its work. "That changed us," says Knox. "It changed how we were thinking about measurement and being able to measure in the three elements of the Triple Aim." It influenced how Kerwin, Knox, and the other leaders thought about what they were trying to accomplish in a broader context. Engaging in the IHI Triple Aim work, Bellin reached out to learn from many different organizations throughout the world where exciting work was going on around population health and the true determinants of health—not just strictly within the health care system.

"We were blown away by the work that other organizations were doing with populations [organizations] that you would think this concept would have no meaning for," says Knox. "CareOregon in Portland is an HMO directed at the Medicaid population. The work they were doing with that Medicaid population and the work that they were doing with an HMO, leading the Triple Aim theory within provider organizations of all kinds of different ownership and size—we were really just amazed by that." Bellin's leaders were struck as well by provider organizations dealing with very challenging populations in New York City's poorer neighborhoods as well as work in Cincinnati's inner city by Cincinnati Children's Hospital. Hearing about successes in places where the demographics were very challenging gave the Bellin team members confidence that they too could reach out and work with some of the more challenging populations in their region. "It was just totally motivating for us and gave us incredible confidence to continue our work and spread it throughout our entire population," says Knox.

## A Deep Dive for Determinants of Health

By 2011, Knox says, the Triple Aim was "embedded in our psyche and our actions."

There are many determinants of health that cannot be altered by an organization such as Bellin: heredity, gender, employment or marital status, income, and education level. But there are many others that an organization effectively tackling the Triple Aim can influence if it partners with various social and community organizations in delivering effective primary care. These include such powerful determinants as personal habits, including exercise, nutrition, and alcohol, tobacco, and drug use.

Bellin teams were already working with employers to get at many of these determinants as they affected employees, but that left large numbers of people in their area—those who do not work, for example—out of the loop. Thus they launched an intensive effort with the Green Bay schools to reach out to children and their families. They launched an effort with seniors and another targeted at the Medicaid population.

But it may be that the initiative with employers is, at least so far, the most influential work on the key determinants of health. Knox's view is that engaging with employees in the workplace has the potential to get at 80 percent of health determinants among the employee population. And if companies were willing to get engaged in the community—in broader issues concerning the environment, employment, the availability of fresh foods, for example—it would probably be possible to get at environmental or economic determinants as well. "It depends upon the company," he says, "and how they want to get involved or not get involved and some of the broader issues that are driving health."

Bellin has taken on the Triple Aim work with a passion. Bellin's leaders understand their population in detail and have identified the essential drivers of health improvement. "We have done the research on what exists at least in the United States around employer strategies and work and we have put that together and applied it with our own population in a comprehensive model," says Knox. "We see examples of really good work but in a sense fragmented work, and I think we have attempted to, with some degree of success, bring together a comprehensive approach to the health of the population."

It is this comprehensive approach, Knox maintains, that tackles the cost aspect of the Triple Aim:

> You can get low costs on your health plan just shifting a lot of the cost over to the employees and not deal with the causal factors usually related to lifestyle and behavior and people making hard changes. When I say we have invested the resources, we have invested in primary care, we have invested in health coaches, we have invested in fitness centers, we have invested in nutritionists.

> We have invested in the resources that are there to help and support people and hopefully a lot of the gain we are seeing is because we are fundamentally dealing with the root causes.

Bellin is also exploring additional collaborations to get at the determinants of population health by working with a variety of government departments, including local health departments and, in order to focus on public safety, police departments. It is reaching out to environmental groups and working on nutrition issues with grocery stores and restaurants. For example, Van Straten cites the NuVal Nutritional Scoring System, which rates food on a 1 to 100 scale with the healthiest foods getting the highest scores. NuVal, for example, rates steamed green beans at 100 and Famous Amos Chocolate Chip Cookies at 10. The idea is to enable consumers to compare foods as quickly and easily on nutrition as they do on price. On its Web site, NuVal describes its scoring system as taking into account "30-plus nutrients and nutrition factors—the good (protein, calcium, vitamins) and the not-so-good (sugar, sodium, cholesterol). And then it boils it down into a simple, easy-to-use number . . . you can trust to make better decisions about nutrition in just a few seconds."

"This system," says Van Straten, "is influencing local buying and having an impact on the production process of foods to make them healthier. . . . People will be talking about this scoring system and how easy it is, and they don't have to sit there and count the calories and calculate the carbs, and it is great if you think of our chronic health, chronic care population, [such as] diabetics, how easy it is for them."

As Bellin has progressed with its work, it has raced past its competitors in recent years. But those competitors soon took notice of what Bellin was doing and have started to follow in Bellin's footsteps, patterning their care and programs after much of what Bellin is doing. This makes for a more competitive environment and actually benefits the community overall. When one health system is going in this direction it has real power. When all health systems are doing so, however, it can be an order of magnitude more powerful and more influential on the overall health of the community. If these ideas spread, they could make a marked difference in health care in the United States.

## Keys to Doing This Work

- **A defined population.** Clearly define and identify the specific population you want to address.
- **A well-planned design.** Employ a comprehensive framework, such as the total health model.

  Assess the leadership position on health and wellness for the population. (Is it a key strategy? Is it discussed regularly? Are measures in place?)

  Assess the health and wellness culture for the population.

  Conduct a deep analysis of the population to gain knowledge for improvement.

  Define the key resources and services available to the population that support health and wellness and that promote lifestyle and behavioral change.

  Define and assess productivity of the population and develop interventions.

  Define a navigation system appropriate to the population to make it easy to access the right care at the right time for the lowest cost.

- **A reliable approach to plan execution.** Develop a structured and disciplined approach to executing on the design or model for the defined population.

  Clearly define the aims.

  Clearly define the measures.

  Use a systemwide improvement model.

# 6

# The Patient and Family Centered Care Methodology and Practice

## *Improving Patient Experience and Clinical Outcomes*

In our aging yet still active population, total joint replacements have become one of the leading Medicare expenditures. In 2010 in the United States, there were 900,000 total joint replacements—600,000 knees and 300,000 hips—at a cost of $4.8 billion. The number of patients needing such replacements is approaching what Dr. Anthony DiGioia calls "epidemic" levels, and it is expected that demand will increase exponentially in the years ahead. DiGioia is a pioneer in developing new technology for such surgery. In his Pittsburgh practice he performs hundreds of such procedures each year. More than that, though, DiGioia is an innovator who has created a new approach to treating patients, not only in orthopedics but in numerous other care experiences as well.

In this chapter, rather than writing about a large institution, we focus on the work of an individual and his team. The essence of DiGioia's work is his determined effort to solve one of the most challenging and pressing problems in health care today: its lack of patient centeredness.

As we have described in other chapters, the 2001 publication of the Institute of Medicine (IOM) report *Crossing the Quality Chasm: A New Health System for the 21st Century* famously listed six elements defining quality care: safe, effective, patient centered, timely, efficient, and equitable. DiGioia believes that when health care focuses intensively on the patient-centered element, the rest of these elements naturally follow. He created a methodology he termed the Patient and Family Centered Care (PFCC) Methodology and Practice to remedy the lack of patient centeredness.

The PFCC Methodology and Practice is predicated on the belief that there is more than enough capacity in the system as it is; that there is no need for any additional resources or spending. The method depends not on new resources but on refocusing existing resources. DiGioia says the work to date—after six years of implementation in more than thirty-three care areas—proves that it enables providers to do more with less. Using the PFCC method, he says, "we can achieve the Triple Aim."

The following 2010 data for patients having hip or knee replacements illustrate the methodology's impressive results (national data are from the Agency for Healthcare Research and Quality):

- The average length of stay at DiGioia's facility for a total knee replacement was 2.9 days, versus the national average of 3.8 days.
- For hip replacements the average length of stay was 2.5 days, versus 4.9 days for the national average.
- Among DiGioia's patients an amazing 92 percent were discharged directly from hospital to home, whereas the national average was 23 to 29 percent.
- Among DiGioia's patients, 99 percent reported that pain was not an impediment to physical therapy, including day-of-surgery physical therapy.
- DiGioia's Press Ganey and HCAHPS (Hospital Consumer Assessment of Healthcare Providers and Systems) mean satisfaction scores (measured in terms of patients who would "refer family and/or friends") were in the 99th percentile nationally.

DiGioia's work indicates that a relentless focus on patients and families yields impressive results on all three aspects of the Triple Aim. Focusing on the cost of care metric alone, it is clear that the PFCC Methodology and Practice approach—by cutting hospital stays nearly in half—has a profound impact.

## Bridging the Gap Between Engineers and Surgeons

Tony DiGioia's interest in the mechanics of the human body was quite personal back in the late 1970s when, as a tight end for the Carnegie Mellon University football team, he suffered a knee injury that sidelined him for the final few games of his freshman season. Fortunately, the MCL (medial collateral ligament) strain did not require surgery, and with time and rehab he was back in action the following year. At the time DiGioia had no sense that he would become one of the nation's leading experts on the very joint he had injured. That would have seemed particularly improbable given his passion for civil engineering, his college major.

He was the oldest of eight children in a Pittsburgh family and he wanted to follow in the footsteps of his dad, a PhD in civil engineering. At Carnegie Mellon DiGioia thrived in the precision of the engineering environment. Upon graduation he advanced to a Carnegie master's degree program in biomedical engineering and worked in an orthopedic biomechanics laboratory doing structural analysis of joints. "On the computer, you could see how a joint replacement would react under certain conditions even before the device was used in a real patient," he says.

As a graduate student he was fortunate to work under the supervision of Dr. Albert Ferguson, a respected orthopedic surgeon. Even in the 1970s and early 1980s, Ferguson understood the importance of bringing in other disciplines—especially engineering—to solve problems in medicine. DiGioia collaborated with residents and other physicians on engineering challenges in orthopedics. He was soon in the habit of attending grand rounds with the residents, and Ferguson encouraged him to consider a career in medicine. Pursuing that idea DiGioia applied and was admitted to Harvard Medical School and headed to Boston, bringing with him Ferguson's counsel that he always try to "bridge the gap between surgeons and engineers."

After an internship in general surgery and a residency in orthopedic surgery at the University of Pittsburgh Medical Center (UPMC), he returned to Boston for a one-year fellowship in adult reconstructive surgery at Massachusetts General Hospital, where he focused largely on hip and knee replacements. After completing his training in 1992, DiGioia headed home to Pittsburgh and joined an orthopedic practice at Shadyside Hospital, which later became part of the UPMC system. At the same time he did something highly unusual for a young surgeon: He started a research lab where he pulled together an interdisciplinary team of engineers and computer experts from Carnegie Mellon to advance the science of orthopedic surgery.

Initially DiGioia and his research team focused on joint replacement computer simulations as a way to plan for surgery. At the time, the science of robotics was developing rapidly, and Carnegie Mellon was one of the leaders in the field. DiGioia and his team eventually combined robotics with computer-assisted surgical tools. To advance their work they received one of the first National Science Foundation grants in medical robotics. DiGioia and his team figured out how to use robotics as a navigation tool, creating what DiGioia describes as "a GPS system for surgeons." It proved to be a breakthrough. Robotics and computer-assisted tools allowed for a more precise alignment of an implant. "Better alignment means fewer problems with wear or dislocations," says DiGioia. "To be able to reproduce the technique with such precision meant consistently better outcomes for all patients. It reduces variation and tightens the best practice."

## Helping to Lead the Way

DiGioia was young, smart, and different. He wanted to build a successful orthopedic surgical practice, but he also wanted to research and innovate. This was unusual and not received entirely well by the other doctors in the practice. After just a year, DiGioia broke out on his own, starting a solo practice. "The best situation for me is when I am helping to lead the way," he says. "When I am in a situation where I don't have an opportunity to lead the way and have an impact on clinical practice, I don't get as excited. It became clear that to continue to be able to do the things I enjoy and want to do and that I felt were my strength, I would have to start my own practice from scratch, and that is what I did."

While in solo practice he worked with others to organize a conference on computer-assisted orthopedic surgery. They dubbed the conference CAOS, and the subsequently formed organization was named CAOS-International (The International Society for Computer Assisted Orthopaedic Surgery). The CAOS conferences commenced in 1995 with a session in Pittsburgh and another in Switzerland, and DiGioia continued to run them for another decade. The meetings were an opportunity to bring together surgeons, engineers, and other scientists who were in the vanguard of computer-assisted surgery.

In the early 2000s, his practice steadily grew and soon several additional surgeons began working in his joint care center at Western Pennsylvania Hospital in the West Penn Allegheny Health System, the first focused care center in western Pennsylvania for patients needing hip and knee replacements.

As central to his professional life as technology had always been, however, he was about to learn something that would open his mind to the possibilities of improvements as no technology ever had.

## Focusing on the *Entire* Care Experience

In the early 2000s, DiGioia realized that for all his focus on technology, the places with the best and most reproducible outcomes "were the ones looking at the entire care experience and not just the surgery. How do you best prepare a patient for surgery? How do you most effectively do pre-op testing? And when? What kind of anesthesia regimen works best? What is the most effective pain management? What is the most successful rapid rehab? How do you get the physical therapists all on the same page? How do you follow up with the patient?"

He reflected on these and other questions over time and realized that he had never before been so clear on the need to focus on the *entire patient experience*. The more he thought about it, the clearer it became. And along with that clarity came his belief that it was also essential to include the patient's family in every step of the process because he could see that family members played an enormous role in a patient's life—before, during, and after treatment.

DiGioia had always prided himself on cross-discipline collaboration, and yet he now realized that he had been working within "a computer-assisted orthopedic surgery silo." He was very much an innovator on the technology side, but he could now see he was otherwise quite traditional. Like most surgeons he viewed the surgical process through a narrow prism, seeing the actual operation itself as *the* event, with everything else as ancillary. But he now saw it differently—that rehab, for example, was just as important to a quality outcome as an accurate surgical technique and that pain management was essential to effective rehabilitation. Some surgeons, perhaps many, dismissed the process pieces—the elements other than the surgery itself—as peripheral, preferring instead to focus on an approach where the skill of the surgeon or the implant design trumped all.

"You had to look at the whole patient experience," DiGioia says. "Traditionally, if you are a surgeon, you are very, very focused on the surgery you perform. We found out that yes, the technique is important, but most times the biggest impact on outcomes was *everything else*." DiGioia saw that a broader approach was more effective. Improving "the patient experience or flow through the whole system and a full cycle of care improved outcomes more than any single technology had and it did so for a greater number of patients."

DiGioia "broke out of that silo" and eagerly embarked on breaking down other silos that prevented developing complete care teams. "There were people out there doing fantastic stuff with process. One group was doing a unique rapid rehab program. Another had developed very progressive pain management techniques. Another was doing unique spinal anesthesia techniques and another had new surgical techniques. There were all these pockets. But *very few had put it all together*." DiGioia went at putting it together with a sense of rejuvenation. He is an intellectual sponge who considers himself an "integrator"; someone who collects information and ideas from others and puts them toward solving clinical challenges such as pre-op planning and procedures, pain management, anesthesia, rehab—every step in the care process through a full cycle of care.

When he referred to "process" and "patient experience," DiGioia meant everything beyond the surgery itself, and it all had to be mapped out. Traditionally, the view in orthopedics had been that there is a pre-op process, then the surgery, then post-op—and that they were all separate pieces. But "from the patient and family perspective, this is a whole experience and you can't separate the pieces," DiGioia says. "If you really want to maximize outcomes, quality, safety, and even efficiencies, you have to look at all the components in the care delivery process."

In August 2006, DiGioia defined in writing, partly in his own shorthand, the problem he sought to solve: "The traditional operating approach in American hospitals is broken and can't be fixed by simply working harder and faster. Fundamental structural problems of current system[s] over-compartmentalize, over-specialize and rely on only one operating approach for all patients. A majority of hospitals center operations on meeting the needs of departments and disciplines rather than patients."

His solution was to examine all processes from a patient's perspective. DiGioia was very much aware that patient-centered care had been a subject in the literature for some years, that the IOM had promoted the importance of patient-centered care and included it as one of the six elements of quality, and that he certainly was not alone in his thinking. Increasing numbers of scholars were recognizing the value of patient-centered care. For example, Guterman et al. (2011) wrote in a Commonwealth Fund report that "within the United States, we have evidence that reorganizing care around the patient with teams that are accountable to each other and to patients and are supported by information systems that guide and drive improvement, has the potential to eliminate waste, reduce medical errors, and improve outcomes—at lower total cost."

An IHI course description on patient experience stated:

> According to new research, the patient experience is one of the top three priorities of hospital leaders over the next three years. It is clearly time to refocus on the person at the center of care. Many

organizations are struggling to understand what patient-centered care truly means, and what it really looks like. Everyone has a role in the patient journey: from the arrivals parking attendant, to the CEO and clinical staff, including environmental services and the check-out receptionist. Successful hospitals provide an exceptional patient experience. Organizations with a culture that focuses on patients are rewarded with higher clinical quality and efficiency, a safer patient environment, greater employee engagement, and improved financial results.

By putting the emphasis on a patient's care experience—including respect, partnership, shared decision making, well-coordinated transitions, and efficiency—hospitals see improvements in their patient satisfaction survey data and HCAHPS. Because HCAHPS scores are publicly available, hospitals scoring high on them can attract more patients, providers, and payers.

The more DiGioia thought about this holistic approach, the more firmly he embedded it into his practice. "Every industry must listen to the end user," he says. "No industry that has survived has failed to focus on the end user. And in health care we don't do that. The industry cannot survive in the current model if we follow a path where we do not listen to the end user and engage them in the design of new approaches. You can't go wrong with a focus on patients and families. You just can't."

## Seeing Something Different About DiGioia's Patients

Notably, even before he began to formally concentrate on patient-centered care, DiGioia was already spontaneously paying closer attention to patients' welfare than many other doctors did. Gigi Conti Crowley, for example, could see that there was something different in the way DiGioia dealt with his patients. As a nurse at Shadyside Hospital, Crowley had an opportunity to observe the way in which many different surgeons dealt with patients. Over time, she noticed that DiGioia's patients would come in for their surgery prepared and knowledgeable about the course of treatment; that they knew about pain management medication and the rehab process and all the other details involved in their treatment. She could see that his patients were clearly better prepared than patients of other surgeons. She also noticed that when DiGioia's patients were discharged, they left the hospital with a clear sense of what the path going forward would be— medications, rehab, follow-up visits, and more. Often she found that patients of other doctors were confused and uncertain. Some would be surprised when she told them they were going home that day. "I would notice and think about his patients," she says. "Why are they so prepared? Everybody was on the same page."

Later he was to communicate this attentiveness to his entire team. "Tony realized that a surgeon is only one part of the whole experience," says Leslie Davis, president of Magee-Womens Hospital of UPMC. "He doesn't try and be more than the one piece. There are many practices where the doctor is really well-meaning—'if you have any pain give me a call and we'll take care of it.' But then when the patient calls, the doctor is in Colorado skiing. Tony realized that he's one piece of the team and he's got to have a team and he has to educate patient as to whose role is for what. All the staff members know their roles. For the staff, it is a very empowering place to be. They can help the patient and it's not just, 'Let's track down Dr. DiGioia.'"

## Designing a New Approach

Around 2005, it became clear to DiGioia that gradually he and his team had revamped the process surrounding surgery and that the newly evolved method—designed from the patient's and family's point of view—was more effective than the traditional approach. He described it as a "low-technology, systems-based approach" to improvement—"the redesign of patient experiences so resources and personnel are organized around patients, rather than around specialized departments and practitioners in a hospital, and through the full cycle of care."

DiGioia began calling this new method the Patient and Family Centered Care (PFCC) Methodology and Practice. This approach encompassed many things, including improved preparation of patients and families prior to surgery. It meant patients fully understanding the alternatives to surgery when such options existed; it meant patients who had no real choice other than surgery understanding the entire process and their active role in it; it meant patients selecting and working side by side with a coach—a spouse, another family member, or a friend—who would assist the patient throughout the entire process. It meant better anesthesia techniques, more innovative and effective pain management, and rapid rehabilitation. It meant engaging with physical therapists from the start to understand the PT path ahead. It meant the use of *focused care teams*, whom DiGioia defined as "health care professionals who work together and specialize in these areas through a full cycle of care"—with equal emphasis on working together (teamwork) and on specializing. The teams typically include doctors, nurses, and medical assistants, but they can also reach far beyond the usual clinical team members to include any person who touches the patient at any time during his or her care experience.

An example of the changes brought about by the new approach involves presurgical testing. Prior to the inception of the Patient and Family Centered Care approach, patients were at the mercy of the traditional hospital approach to preparation prior to surgery. They were moved from department to department for various tests, such as blood work, chest X-rays, EKGs, and more. This could take several hours and meant a great deal of scheduling and coordination of appointments that the patients had to arrange themselves.

The PFCC approach established a one-stop-shop approach to these requirements by setting up a center for joint replacement patients only. "Instead of sending patients to various departments for tests, we brought the testing to them," says DiGioia. Patients and their coaches went to the clinic for a focused, sixty- to ninety-minute session during which they received all the required testing and focused, comprehensive education.

The Patient and Family Centered Care Methodology and Practice embodied DiGioia's belief that innovation happened when people from different disciplines collaborated. "One of the basic tenets of the PFCC Methodology is that we bring together people who work within the walls of the same facility but may have never worked together before," he says. "Because we focus on the patient and family throughout the care experience, it is important to work hand in hand with the parking attendant and the physician and dietary and nursing—to bring *all* the caregivers together."

DiGioia knew, for example, how important it was that patients arrive for their first pre-op meeting and their day of surgery feeling as focused and unstressed as possible. The calmer and more focused they were, the more they would learn and the more effectively they would engage. Yet DiGioia and his team learned from patient feedback that the experience of arriving at the hospital and not knowing where to park and not being certain exactly which entrance to use caused stress even before they entered the building! Thus DiGioia and his team revised that process so patients were given precise instructions for exactly where to park and exactly how to get to the office. What's more, DiGioia and his team members engaged the parking attendants, recognizing that because they "touched" the patient experience, they were caregivers. This focus on a patient's ability to park easily is indicative of how seriously the methodology takes each step in the process.

"The parking piece is very important," says DiGioia. "Human nature is that first impressions are important, and the first person you see and deal with at the hospital many times is the parking person. It's important because it sets the stage for the rest of the experience." If a patient arrives and is unable to find a place to park, his or her level of anxiety and frustration rises rapidly. Perhaps the patient will have to walk too far—these are people often coming for knee or hip replacements! Perhaps they will be late. "A lot of it is anxiety reduction," says DiGioia. "Health care itself 99 percent of the time is anxiety provoking—even for a well visit. A patient's mind state affects outcomes. It affects the physiology of the care experience. This isn't just touchy-feely." (And it also affects hospital processes. DiGioia notes that when the day surgery unit at UPMC Presbyterian Hospital applied the PFCC method to the arrival experience of patients, including parking, one result was a reduction in operating room delays, which in turn improved efficiency and productivity.) In an effort to fully understand exactly what patients were experiencing, DiGioia and staff members sat down for conversations, listening to what patients worried about, hoped for, and expected. He also engaged college students, students in the health professions, and caregivers to *shadow* patients and report back on precisely what was happening to them from initial visit through the hospital stay, rehab, and follow-up visits. Patient and family shadowing is the direct, real-time observation of patients and families as they move through each step of a care experience. An entire care experience or segments of an experience can be shadowed. The shadower is charged with seeing the care experience through the eyes of the patient and family and recording all that he or she sees. A shadower is able to

- Observe the steps in the care process as they happen, including how long each step takes.
- Record and understand the patient's and family's reactions to what happens at each step.
- Map the flow of care for patients and families.

The shadowing DiGioia requested produced a comprehensive *care experience flow map*, as DiGioia called it, showing exactly what patients and families went through. This precise picture of the current state then enabled DiGioia and his team to identify waste and inefficiency and to revamp many elements of their process. For example, shadowing and flow mapping identified the following touchpoints and caregivers who would make up the care experience working group.

| Touchpoints | Caregivers |
| --- | --- |
| Initial contact | Parking attendant; physician assistant |
| Office visit | Receptionist; pre-op educator |
| Preoperative education and testing | Medical assistant; pre-op nurse |
| Surgery | Nurse practitioner; anesthesiologist |
| Inpatient stay | Radiology technician; surgeon |
| Discharge | Checkout receptionist; OR team; PACU (postanesthesia care unit) nurse; transport nurse; aide; physical therapist; occupational therapist |

## Magee: Spreading the Method

The more he used, tested, improved, and measured the methodology, the more convinced DiGioia became that it could be spread to other care areas and not used just in orthopedics. He believed that it could be applied to *just about any care experience* and any organization and facility, inpatient or outpatient, to achieve similar results and that it could improve outcomes not only for orthopedic patients but for *all* patients.

But he needed to prove that it would work beyond orthopedics. He needed to be able to take his methodology to a place where he could spread it to dozens of other care experiences and see whether it worked as well as he expected. He had hoped to do this at the West Penn Allegheny Health System where he was then located, but discussions with the hospital's administrative leaders did not lead where he had hoped they would. He needed to be in a place that would embrace the opportunity. This would mean leaving Western Pennsylvania Hospital, where he had been for five years, but DiGioia's loyalty was much more to the methodology he had developed and its potential to improve care than to any clinical location.

In the summer of 2005, DiGioia called an old friend from his days as a resident, Dr. Freddie Fu, who is chief of orthopedics at the University of Pittsburgh Medical Center (UPMC). Fu set up a meeting for himself and DiGioia with Elizabeth Concordia, executive vice president of the UPMC system, and it was clear they wanted DiGioia to join them. He was, after all, a very busy, well-known surgeon who would bring significant revenue into the hospital. But it was more than that.

"I told them flat out that I wasn't interested in moving my practice just to move my practice," he says. "I explained that I wanted to develop demonstration projects to show how this methodology can be applied to *any care experience* and I explained the process. I said, 'It is important to me to have a platform to test, evolve, and spread the methodology as broadly and quickly as possible.' Liz got it right away." Discussions continued with Concordia and her team about how to not only incorporate his practice but also expand and accelerate the spread of the PFCC methodology.

Concordia suggested he bring his team to Magee Womens Hospital, one of twenty-two hospitals in the UPMC system. Magee was a 280-bed facility historically devoted to women's health issues, although it had begun to offer broader services as well. To DiGioia its advantages were many. It did not currently have an orthopedics department, which meant he would be able to develop a program from the ground up. It had an empty floor available, and there was a commitment to provide all the equipment and services he needed to develop a first-class program. Most important was the commitment from Concordia to make the new program a demonstration model for the system.

"People thought we were crazy," he says. "They would say, 'why are you moving to a women's hospital that doesn't even have orthopedics?'" But DiGioia and his team saw it as a great opportunity to take the concept of patient- and family-centered care to the next level. He saw that at Magee he could develop a subspecialty hospital within the walls of an existing hospital—a "hospital within a hospital." Thus was born the Bone and Joint Center at Magee Women's Hospital of UPMC, where DiGioia has been practicing in the new Orthopaedic Program since February 2006. Another part of his efforts at this time was to have the UPMC fund an innovation center to promote spread of the PFCC Methodology and Practice.

## Six Steps from Current State to Ideal Experience

Applying the PFCC Methodology and Practice entails six fairly simple steps that have been defined by DiGioia.

### Step 1

Select a care experience. DiGioia urges caregivers to consider what area is in the greatest need of improvement. What areas do patients and families feel need improvement? In what areas do the institution's HCAHP scores reveal a deficiency? What areas have energetic leaders—men and women with a sense of urgency for change? "Always look for the people with sense of urgency because you will give them everything else they need to make change," DiGioia says.

Also determine whether the focus will be on a complete care experience or a partial care experience. "With orthopedic surgery, for example, you could choose to use the method to improve just the day of surgery for a total joint replacement," DiGioia says. "You can target a whole process or just a piece."

### Step 2

Establish a care experience *guiding council*. The initial participants should be a core team of caregivers determined to improve. They will become the champions of the improvement process. The *administrative champion* (the organization's vice president, COO, or CEO) works to remove administrative barriers, and the *clinical champion* does the same on the clinical side. A PFCC coordinator serves as chief communicator for and from the group. The council meets for thirty to sixty minutes every week in order to drive change and sets the stage of the full-care experience working group.

### Step 3

Evaluate the current state and develop a sense of urgency to drive change. This is what Dr. Gary Kaplan, CEO at Virginia Mason Medical Center, likes to describe as "draining the swamp" in order to see the reality of the current state. There are many ways to determine the current state but one of the most effective involves the shadowing technique DiGioia used to improve orthopedic surgery. "When you shadow a care experience two or three times, it is amazing how the same things come up over and over again," he says. "When you shadow and view everything through the eyes of the patient and their family, people are surprised because they thought they knew the current state."

As described earlier, shadowing also permits caregivers to develop a true and accurate care experience flow map. Drawing a visual map that shows the experience reveals gaps and wasted time and motion. It also reveals opportunities for improvement.

Other tools that help to determine the current state are patient and family advisory councils and storytelling. Patient and family storytelling (defined as any information the team derives from the patient or a family member) brings the voice of the patient directly to the team. Such stories, whether written or, even more powerfully, captured on audio or video recorders, can supplement surveys by allowing patients to explain how they think and feel about their care experience and how it might be improved (video ethnography is discussed in Chapter Seven). The orthopedic *patient and family advisory council* is composed of patients, family members, and caregivers who work as partners in codesigning an exceptional care experience. Yet another tool consists of HCAHP reports, which help to fill in details of the current state, particularly areas of weakness. Although all these tools for getting at the current state have value, DiGioia says that "shadowing and care experience flow mapping are the most important because they identify caregiver touchpoints and highlight bottlenecks and redundancies."

### Step 4

Expand the PFCC guiding council to the full-care experience working group based on the shadowing and care experience flow map caregiver touchpoints. The working group can range from a dozen to two dozen caregivers involved in the care experience of patients and their families. Or, as DiGioia puts it, caregivers who "touch the patient and family in some way." In the PFCC Methodology and Practice approach, caregivers are defined as any individuals in the health care setting whose work touches a patient's or family's experience, including doctors, nurses, therapists, technicians, dietitians, appointment schedulers, parking attendants, janitors, and also individuals that patients and families may never see, such as hospital leaders, supply chain employees, medical records clerks, and financial representatives.

The full-care experience working group membership is determined by the care experience flow map and caregiver touchpoints and is drawn from a wide range of departments, which helps to break down silos. The caregivers invited to participate must come from all departments and all levels of the organization in order to achieve coordination across the traditional care silos. DiGioia strongly suggests that invitations to prospective team members for the critical working group kick-off come in the form of a formal letter from the CEO. This conveys both the importance of the work and the commitment to it from the top of the organization.

The caregivers agree to serve as members of the working group and meet for just one hour each week. Given the power of leadership to effect disruptive change, it is crucial that the hospital's COO or vice president be part of the working group and attend weekly meetings and that the hospital president or CEO also make his or her presence known by participating on a regular basis in the meetings.

At each working group meeting, feedback from patients and families guides the projects the group will focus on. In addition, project improvement leaders report on the status of their active projects.

### Step 5

Create a shared vision of the ideal patient and family care experience by writing the ideal story. This is a wonderful step that allows all the members of the working group and soon-to-be-formed care experience project improvement teams to envision perfection. During this part of the process, there is no limit to what can be imagined—no constraints of resources, time, or anything else. The whole concept is to conjure the best possible patient and family experience and then compare that with the current state.

In February 2007, UPMC Presbyterian Hospital's PFCC day of surgery care experience working group formed. The care experience was defined as running from the time of the office visit to the time a patient was discharged from ambulatory surgery or the inpatient unit. Table 6.1 contains a brief example of the working group's shadowing results (the real story) and segments of the ideal story written by the working group members.

When the working group members set the shadowing results and the ideal story side by side, the question they ask is how can they get from one to the other? How can they make change that will make the current state a thing of the past and replace it with the ideal for patients and families?

### Step 6

Identify potential improvement projects by comparing the current state to the ideal patient experience and get assistance from patients and families in prioritizing these projects. Once projects

**Table 6.1. A Working Group Looks at the Real Experience and Creates an Ideal Experience**

| | Shadowing Results | Ideal Story |
|---|---|---|
| Portal experience | Wayfinding—inadequate directional signage in garage and hospital.<br><br>Patients were parking in three separate parking garages with minimal valet or wheelchair patient assistance available. | "I was handed driving directions and directions were also available on the website for my family and friends. I was also offered the option to have the hospital van pick me up at my home and transport me and my husband to the hospital." |
| Preoperative experience | Anesthesia testing guidelines for surgery were not consistent. Patients were unsure of what testing was needed and why they were sent to the pre-testing department.<br><br>Education materials provided to the patients from the surgeon's office were outdated. | "The surgeon explains the reason for the surgery, the procedure, the risk and benefits of the surgery and why it will help. She provides me with printed information so that I can take it home, read it as often as I need to, and talk with my family about it. My doctor explains that many other materials like this are on the UPMC website for my use at any time. I am handed a booklet and a DVD about the surgical experience and the same-day surgery intake process at the facility where my procedure will take place."<br><br>"My pre-op testing day goes very smoothly and efficiently. I am given an itinerary with each step to be completed in order. Everyone greets me warmly by name and introduces me to the next person whom I have to see." |
| Transport | UPMC Presbyterian is housed in two separate buildings connected by a bridge that is a quarter mile long.<br><br>The walkway was congested, with no designated path for patients being transported. | "My surgery is in the same building as the Family Lounge. I don't have to be transported over any bridges or tunnels, and my husband doesn't have to walk between buildings." |

| | | |
|---|---|---|
| | Most patients were being transported by stretchers whether they were required or not.<br><br>There was one transporter manipulating equipment while pushing the stretcher—this was difficult for the transporter. | |
| Family lounge | The waiting room was outdated, cold, and the seating was uncomfortable.<br><br>The communication between caregivers and families could be improved.<br><br>Pagers were unreliable and overall the environment was noisy.<br><br>The room attendant was yelling pager numbers and family last names for patient updates. | "My husband is given a code number so that he can check my progress on the electronic tracking board without it having to list my name. He stops at the bistro area for a cup of coffee, since we had to leave so early. He has brought a laptop computer and checks his emails using the hospital's free wireless connection. In the Family Lounge there are computer stations. Every two hours a liaison updates him on my progress." |
| Discharge | Discharge instructions were received shortly before patient left.<br><br>Patient and family were unaware of the expected length of stay. | "On the day of surgery the liaison gives me and my husband a 'flight plan' that details my journey throughout the day until my discharge, with expected time estimates specified. She explains that if there are delays, a member of the staff will explain why and will revise the times of the flight plan."<br><br>"My husband is told he can have my discharge prescriptions filled onsite, and he eagerly accepts this opportunity. I feel confident in understanding what is expected when I go home as my entire care team provided clear direction since my first office visit." |

are identified, form PFCC methodology project improvement teams that meet weekly to get the work done, using the techniques and tools mentioned in steps 1 to 5. Focus improvements initially on easy to do, low-tech, low-cost solutions to generate positive results and enthusiasm for the process.

Says DiGioia, "The PFCC Methodology and Practice is a process that has a beginning but has no end; caregivers continually identify whole care experiences as well as smaller segments in need of improvement, make changes following these six steps, evaluate the changes made, make further improvements, evaluate again, and so on in a continual cycle of change and measurement."

"The PFCC process gives the patient comfort," says Gigi Conti Crowley, director of DiGioia's orthopedic program at Magee. "They know exactly what is happening to them and when. They have met all the people they will be dealing with throughout the process—the nurse, scheduler, Dr. DiGioia, the physical therapist. 'I will be the person who greets you on your day of surgery. I will be here with you and we will go through exactly the process I just described.' Already you've reduced their anxiety."

## Identifying the Foundation of PFCC

Anthony DiGioia, Pamela K. Greenhouse, and Timothy J. Levison (2007) have described the series of eight steps that make up the foundation of patient- and family-centered care: "(1) patient and family education; (2) less invasive techniques; (3) multimodal anesthesia and pain management techniques; (4) rapid rehabilitation protocols; (5) rapid outcomes feedback (from the patients' and the providers' perspectives) resulting in efficient program changes; (6) creating a learning environment and culture; (7) developing a sense of community, competition, and team among patients and between patients and caregivers and staff; and (8) promoting a wellness (rather than sickness) approach to recovery."

DiGioia, Greenhouse, and Levison broke the process down into segments, starting with the office visit about three weeks prior to surgery. This visit "is organized as one-stop testing and education to set the stage for hospitalization. The streamlined visit allows patients to complete needed testing and education in approximately two hours. The visit also provides an opportunity to meet other patients and families who will be having surgery at the same time as well as staff." Meeting other patients facing a similar procedure is generally comforting to patients. They see that they are far from alone in the challenge they face. They relax a bit more when engaging with others, and they quite often exchange information and answer one another's questions, thus learning from one another in a beneficial way.

This special pre-op teaching and testing session prepares the patient not only for surgery but for discharge as well. The patient meets in the office with a social worker who provides an overview of the anticipated discharge plan—the release date for going home and the plan for home care. This is a critical piece for it gives the patient a full picture of the process. It is the type of information that enables the patient to assemble all the pieces in his or her mind and gain a sense of calm and control by being well informed. Also, understanding the full spectrum of care enables a patient to think through the process and identify any gaps to ask questions about. The better informed the patient is from the start, the sharper and more useful the questions he or she is able to ask. The patient and staff also preschedule the first post-op visit as well, which completes the full cycle of the care experience from the patient's and family's perspective.

An additional crucial piece of the process comes with the selection of a coach for the patient—typically a family member or close friend. The coach, DiGioia et al.(2007) write, "will help the patient in the postsurgical recovery phase of his or her joint replacement and provides a single point of contact and communication among healthcare providers, patients, and other family members." DiGioia adds that "families and coaches are caregivers who are free and willing to help, but we have not fully tapped into this resource."

On the day of the surgery the physician is thinking about the patient, as opposed to just the surgery. During a brief reassuring discussion prior to surgery, the surgeon may answer any last-minute questions from either patient or coach and will seek to reassure and calm both. The surgeon also—with both coach and patient observing—marks the site of the surgery.

After talking with the surgeon, patient and coach gather with the anesthesiologist "and learn more about special anesthesia techniques and postoperative pain management options. Anesthesia emphasis is on managing patient expectations; multimodal pain management protocols; integrating pre-, intra-, and postoperative care; the relation between pain and nausea treatment; and a commitment to low-cost pain management."

When the patient enters the OR for the procedure, he or she is surrounded by seasoned clinical experts whose professional lives are focused on total joint replacement operations. The team consists of specialists in their areas—from the surgeon to the nurses to the operating room staff. The result of all the preparation and the expertise of the staff is, as DiGioia et al. write, "standardization, which reduces variability and improves quality, reduces down time, improves productivity, reduces stress for the surgeon and operating room staff, and leads to reproducible results. Dedicated staff and reduction in variability necessarily mean enhanced skill development of the entire team. Speed is not synonymous with efficiency, but rather a byproduct of these combined results."

When surgery is complete and patients are returned to their hospital rooms, they dress in street clothes to get ready for the rehabilitation process, which begins within hours, as pain management enables patients to get up, move around, and begin the types of exercise that will hasten their healing process.

One of the most attractive aspects of the PFCC methodology— particularly appealing to hospital administrators and caregivers alike—is its simplicity. It is quite different from having someone come in and saying we believe you should shift your management system over to Six Sigma or the Toyota Production System. Such vast changes, although ideal for some provider organizations, are not a fit for others.

The PFCC methodology, in contrast, says DiGioia, "is simple, intuitive and it gets people focused. If you focus on the right thing, everything else falls into place. These are very simple solutions for very complicated patient flow processes and disease states. In health care we tend to make things so complicated. This is such a simple approach. It's really commonsense simple solutions. And in complex systems, simple solutions are the best."

## Spreading PFCC to Other Care Experiences

Although the PFCC Methodology and Practice is simple and flexible, it requires the presence of certain elements, and as is so often the case in any industry, the central ingredient is leadership. Although it is critical to have frontline workers embrace the method, it is equally critical to have administrative and clinical leaders embrace it. "Chances of success for disruptive or transformational processes significantly improve if you have CEO support," DiGioia says. "It takes hold much faster if you have a champion."

DiGioia's experience is that *evangelists*, who might make up no more than 5 percent of a workforce, are the ones who drive change. That experience is supported by "studies of organizational development from John Kotter's and Clayton Christiansen's books," says DiGioia. "They both indicate that it is very common in a complex system that an individual might feel that they cannot do anything to change the culture—that it seems overwhelming to get ten thousand employees to think in a new way. But you don't need 100 percent buy in. If you have true evangelists, the early adopters with a passion for the change, you can make it happen, especially if you have the support of the CEO. With support from [the 5 percent who are] evangelists you are in a very good position to change the culture in your organization."

The first place the PFCC Methodology and Practice was spread to after the Orthopaedic Program began was the Women's Cancer Program at Magee. "We wanted to see if we could make PFCC work outside of the ortho realm," says Judy Herstine, the administrator of the Women's Cancer Program. "We wanted to see if it would work in an existing service line with lots of different physicians in lots of different areas." Herstine became a champion for the new work and assembled a team that included representatives from breast surgery, radiation and medical oncology, radiology, nursing, outpatient services, and more. The team gathered together with a half dozen patients to talk informally and listen and learn from what was on the patients' minds.

"One of the big things was how long it took once a patient had an abnormal mammogram to get to biopsy to definitely determine is it cancer or is it not cancer," says Herstine. "We always struggled to decrease that time. It was such an anxious time for women—until the physicians in the room heard the patients talk about how much that time affected them. Their reaction was, 'Wow, we've always been insistent that the breast program focus around efficiency for our most limited resource—a radiologist. How do we make the radiologist most productive? It's always been set up so that it is the most efficient way *for the radiologist*.'" They made an immediate change enabling patients to get a biopsy the same day as they had the mammogram, and they went from an average wait for the results from two weeks to a single day. In the course of the PFCC work, Herstine says the team also identified fifteen to twenty other areas of significance to patients where "we weren't doing as good a job as we should."

Elizabeth Concordia says one of the advantages to the method is that there are few barriers to it. Once it is introduced to a hospital department and people in other areas of the hospital see its impact, "it becomes almost like a snowball effect because it spreads itself."

Nevertheless, as with almost any significant change in health care, there were barriers. One obstacle in particular to spreading the PFCC methodology was that many clinicians would insist that they were already patient focused and always had been. But a closer examination, via shadowing and care experience flow mapping, would often reveal that their structure was not as patient focused as they thought—and in some cases not even close.

Sometimes skeptics could be persuaded by the idea that DiGioia had drawn on one of the leading change authorities in academia. Harvard Business School professor John Kotter had been writing about change management for decades, and DiGioia drew guidance and inspiration from Kotter's 1996 book *Leading Change* and its eight-step change process. DiGioia has read and studied widely among some of the leading theorists on process, economics, and management in health care. From Kotter he learned how to change organizations and the sense of urgency needed to drive change. From *Redefining Health Care* by Michael Porter and Elizabeth Teisberg (2006), DiGioia learned about the concept of value in health care. From Regina Herzlinger's *Market-driven Health Care: Who Wins, Who Loses in the Transformation of America's Largest Service Industry* (1997), he read about focused care centers and viewing care from the patient's perspective. "She calls it consumer-driven health care, but it really is viewing care from the end user and supports codesign," he says. From Clayton Christensen, author of *The Innovator's Dilemma: When New Technologies Cause Great Firms to Fall* (1997), DiGioia came to understand PFCC as a disruptive process and how to introduce disruptive processes into an organization.

## Spreading PFCC to Trauma Care

Obstacles were also encountered when Concordia wanted to implement the PFCC Methodology and Practice in the trauma unit at UPMC's Presbyterian Hospital. Dr. Lou Alarcon, the trauma program director, was reluctant. The department, one of the busiest among any in the UPMC chain, cares for five thousand challenging patients per year—upward of half of them surgical patients. Ninety percent of the patients suffer from blunt trauma such as head injuries and fractures, many of them from falls or car crashes. The work is intense, fast paced, and pressure packed. The trauma team is in the business of evaluating patients very quickly, in most cases operating on them, and focusing on little other than keeping the patient alive.

"When I first heard about PFCC I was skeptical," says Alarcon. "I thought it would take up too much time, more meetings, interfere with the care of patients, cost money. I knew PFCC had worked great for Tony in elective orthopedic surgery, but I didn't think it could be applied to trauma patients. It sounded fluffy and we surgeons are not the most touchy-feely."

But as Alarcon learned more, he saw enough merit to be willing to give it a try. Alarcon met weekly with a team that included "anyone in trauma we thought could potentially interact with the patient or family—nurses, techs, cafeteria people, clergy." Interns shadowed trauma patients in the ensuing weeks and months, following them from the moment they entered the trauma unit until they were released. "We wanted to see the entire experience from their perspective," Alarcon says.

An example of one fairly modest change—but a change very important to patients—involved cervical collars. The standard practice in the trauma unit was to immediately apply a cervical collar as a precaution, and those collars typically remained on patients for twenty-four hours or more until they had a CT scan to make sure there was no neck injury. "The collars are not only very uncomfortable, they can also cause pressure sores and might impair the ability to clear an airway," Alarcon says. "Patients had always complained about them and were very eager to get them off. But it was a very low priority for us." By focusing on the issue, however, the team found a relatively simple way to get radiologists to read the scans within thirty minutes and promptly get the collars off the majority of patients right then. "We realized after we achieved this that it was budget neutral and just required us to identify things that mattered to the patient," says Alarcon.

The trauma team also created a volunteer concierge service so that when family members arrive, personnel are available to get them to their loved one quickly and to help them navigate the system.

Historically, when a patient complained the trauma unit team would react. "But now we're more proactive, not waiting for a complaint," says Alarcon. "We're trying to create a culture where we *always* see things from the perspective of the patient and family."

After adopting the PFCC Methodology and Practice, Alarcon and his team made a significant discovery. In the course of shadowing returning patients who were visiting the ambulatory clinic for follow-up care, the team found that a significant number of trauma patients were developing post-traumatic stress disorder (PTSD) after being released from the hospital. Often in the past patients had suffered debilitating depression, yet because the trauma unit team had been unaware of this, nothing had been done to try to help these patients psychologically. With this new discovery, however, the team began to screen all trauma patients to try to identify those at risk for PTSD and found about 25 percent of patients testing positive for PTSD symptoms. "That's a huge number affected in their ability to interact with their families, to work, everything in their lives," says Alarcon.

Now, those testing positive are counseled by trained nurses and in some cases referred to specialists for treatment. The whole PFCC methodology experience has been "eye-opening" for the trauma unit, says Alarcon. "You could think this is fluff, but when you engage the patient and put patient at the center of the process with tools to make informed decisions, the outcomes are better."

As a result of the team's work, Press Ganey patient satisfaction scores have risen from 77 to 87 percent in the emergency department and from 70 to 80 percent in the general trauma inpatient unit. In addition, in early 2010, staff turnover in trauma areas, including the emergency department, was found to have declined from 35 percent to 12 percent over the previous two years.

And finally, lost patient belongings in the trauma areas have declined from as many as twenty-five individual bags of possessions per week to zero. In the scheme of things this last statistic may not seem particularly significant, but when people are literally traumatized by injury, losing their most important personal possessions serves only to increase their stress at a time when the very last thing that will promote their healing and well-being is additional stress.

Concordia has found the PFCC method "easy to adapt because you are engaging the frontline people who work in that area and it's sustainable. It's not a consultant coming in and leaving. The people there are making the changes. When you use a consultant from the outside, . . . [once he or she leaves] many times things go back to the way they were." When Concordia talks about PFCC she emphasizes that it changes culture, delivers quality outcomes, and is sustainable. "The outcome is an ideal patient experience," she says.

## Results

Thus far the PFCC Methodology and Practice has been spread to more than thirty varied care experiences at numerous UPMC hospitals. It has been implemented in doctor's offices, outpatient facilities, as well as various kinds of hospitals—large and small, tertiary to community, and specialty to teaching.

"By refocusing existing resources and using the tools and techniques of the PFCC Methodology and Practice, we break down silos between departments," says DiGioia. "We maintain an unwavering focus on seeing the care experience through the eyes of patients and families, and achieve measurable improvements in patient satisfaction, caregiver satisfaction, and cost savings for the organization."

The PFCC Methodology and Practice affects the cost of care in a number of ways, including by focusing on reducing waste and inefficiency in the delivery of care. The key is an acute awareness of every step in the care process and identifying which steps most effectively serve patients. Anything that is not value added for the patient is eliminated. The team-based nature of the methodology plays an important role in waste reduction. The focus on every step in the care process results in improved outcomes and reduced complications and readmissions. The fact that DiGioia's patients spend significantly less time in the hospital than the national average for such patients has a huge impact on cost savings and quality, partly because home is a much safer environment than a hospital.

The outcomes of the Orthopaedic Program at Magee-Womens Hospital of UPMC are a reflection of the patient and family care focus. In 2010, the Orthopaedic Program performed 1,551 total knee and total hip replacement (primary and revision) procedures, which included 626 primary knee replacement and 412 primary hip replacement procedures. We began this chapter by pointing out DiGioia's high Press Ganey and HCAHP scores, and how quickly DiGioia's patients were able to go home (after 2.9 days for knee replacement patients compared to 3.8 days nationally and after 2.5 days for hip replacement patients compared to 4.9 days nationally). In addition, 91 percent of knee patients and 92 percent of hip patients were able to go directly home following surgery, compared to national averages of 23 to 29 percent. Going directly home following surgery is important as it has been shown to be associated with lower postoperative complications and also with greater independence in walking, climbing stairs, and getting into and out of bed and chairs. Other outcomes are also impressive:

- Infection rates for the Orthopaedic Program were 0.3 percent for total knee replacements and 0.7 percent for total hip replacements, compared to the national infection rate average of 2.4 percent for knees and 1.7 percent for hips.

- The Orthopaedic Program's inpatient mortality rate was 0 percent for both total knee replacement and total hip replacement patients.
- Readmission rates:

| Readmissions in 2010 | Percentage of All Patients |
| --- | --- |
| Within 30 days | 1.5 |
| Within 60 days | 0.6 |
| Within 90 days | 0.0 |

- On average, only 6 percent of primary total hip or knee replacement patients received transfusions.

DiGioia is "convinced that the outcomes that our patients have are much better . . . [owing to] the combination of techniques, implants, but most importantly, process."

As the Patient and Family Centered Care Methodology and Practice spreads through the UPMC system, the improved patient outcomes are having direct financial results.

For example, a *Health Affairs* article on DiGioia's PFCC work found that "unpublished data show that 272 of the 743 elective spine surgery patients at UPMC Presbyterian Hospital admitted in 2010 were discharged ahead of schedule, and 312 were released on schedule, saving a total of 336 hospital days and $117,600. Average length-of-stay in 2010 decreased by 0.87 days for spine surgery patients compared with 2008," before Presbyterian Hospital adopted the Patient and Family Centered Care approach (Meyer, 2011). An additional financial impact is the competitive advantage that results for hospitals that adopt PFCC-related improvements. When patients learn about the quality metrics at Magee, for example, they are more likely to have their surgery done there than elsewhere.

DiGioia contends that another financial benefit is the cost savings that come with increased staff satisfaction as the engagement and partnerships with patients and families fostered by the PFCC methodology "returns us to our core mission as caregivers." And a paper written for the Innovation Center of UPMC by DiGioia and his colleagues makes the case that patient satisfaction also leads to better profitability:

Many health care leaders find it difficult to make a direct correlation between patient satisfaction and profitability. However,
organizations such as Press Ganey, Gallup, Planetree and the
Healthcare Financial Management Association are increasingly
showing the importance of the relationship between patient
satisfaction and profitability.

A recent article published by the Healthcare Financial Management Association shows that hospitals with consistently high levels
of patient satisfaction are the same hospitals that are among
the most fiscally successful. . . . [A] research study conducted by
Press Ganey . . . demonstrates the correlation between patient
satisfaction and hospital profitability [PFCC Partners of UPMC,
2008, see fig. 3 for the Press Ganey findings].

DiGioia bolsters the case that the PFCC approach controls
costs by citing the fact that since the extension of the PFCC
Methodology and Practice to more than three dozen care experiences not a single new hire has been necessary to implement the
methodology. Relying on existing resources, a variety of clinical
areas have improved outcomes, quality, and safety while reducing
waste and improving the quality of care.

DiGioia also says that no additional personnel have been
necessary for carrying out the process of applying the PFCC
method. Every group applying the method has found ways to
refocus existing personnel to streamline and improve the care
experience.

## Teaching and Spreading the Method Far Beyond UPMC

One wintry day in 2011, DiGioia stood in front of a gathering in
Pittsburgh—a group of providers from throughout the United
States and from other countries as far away as Qatar. They had
convened to learn the PFCC Methodology and Practice. Wearing
a button-down shirt, DiGioia spoke in an easy, comfortable manner. He had never met most of these people before, but he knew
what they were going through and he understood their frustrations and aspirations. *He knew what they wanted for their patients
and families!* And he wanted to introduce them to the PFCC

Methodology and Practice in the hope that they would take it back home and implement it. He was explicit in stating that the most important way to measure the adaptability and simplicity of the method was by getting a positive answer to the question: Can you take this home to your practice or hospital and apply it? Finally, he was not at all bashful about stating his ambition for the PFCC approach. "We don't want little pockets of success," he said. "We want acceleration and widespread adoption."

Providers everywhere have been looking at the current state of care in their hospitals or physician practices and knowing that they could do better; that patients deserve better; that quality and efficiency improvements are within reach. But when they have contrasted the current state with their vision of the ideal state they have often stumbled.

"There is no right answer for every organization," says DiGioia.

> There is a range of ways to engage families and patients. With the PFCC method and the codesign process that is inherent to the approach, *you* decide what is best for *your* patients and families at *your* place with the help of patients and families as partners. We are not saying we have the exact solution to all your problems but we have a *methodology* for you to get there. When you tell people you have the solution to their problems, it turns them off. What we're saying is that you are going to solve the problems at your own place because you understand those issues and circumstances intimately. What we can do is provide the tools to get there. That's what the PFCC Methodology and Practice is all about.

## Keys to Doing This Work

- Focus on the care experience including transitions of care and communications through a full cycle of care.
- View all care as an experience through the eyes of patients and families.
- Conduct shadowing and care experience flow mapping to see the needs of the patient and family as well as the path of the care journey and possible barriers. The new way to see will inspire innovative ideas and new ways to care for patients across the continuum of care.

- Design for the population. With the vision of the patient's journey in hand, design for the entire experience, from diagnosis through treatment, until the patient has recovered to full functionality.
- Teamwork. Invite all who interact with patients to join in the design process. The care processes will produce better outcomes, delightful patient and team experiences at a lower cost, and the additional benefit is strong and effective teams.
- Use the methodology to produce new designs without bringing in additional resources.
- Caregivers partner with patients and families in codesigning care delivery with patients and families.
- Apply PFCC to any care experience to go from your current state to the ideal.

# 7

# Kaiser Permanente

## *Embedding Improvement Capacity into Organizational DNA*

How does one describe a health care organization with 167,000 employees, 16,000 doctors, 593 ambulatory care clinics, 37 medical centers, and nearly 9 million members spread out over eight regions? Through the years we have come to know Kaiser Permanente (KP) well. Although KP is a massive organization, it has proven over time to be both nimble and highly innovative. In fact, it deserves to be counted among the most effective innovators anywhere in health care—which is why we have chosen KP to anchor our book of innovators.

The consensus in our country that the current health care pathway is unsustainable leads us in search of a new way forward. That new pathway may bear a striking resemblance to KP's integrated approach, which aligns the interests of all stakeholders—patients, providers, communities, and those who pay the bills for health care services. KP shows new ways of doing an array of things in health care and we describe some compelling examples of the work in this chapter—work that gets at broad, sweeping issues as well as work that bores into some of the most intractable challenges at the very front lines of care. It is work that improves the health of populations, enhances the patient experience of care, and aims to control the cost of care.

An important component of this work is KP's internal capacity to spread innovations and improvements. Even though a culture of innovation creates a fertile environment in which to improve, great ideas don't do much good unless they are effectively spread and applied in a sustained way at the front lines of care. Some organizations are highly competent at this, but many in health care are not. Although KP is vastly larger than almost every other provider organization in the United States, many of its tools and techniques for spreading and sustaining improvement can be adopted by providers of almost any size.

Perhaps as much as anything else, the story of KP is the *institutional leadership* it provides for the rest of the health care industry in the United States and beyond. By doing what it does in so many realms, KP embodies a better way in pursuit of the Triple Aim.

## World-Class Technology to Improve Health

Technology is an essential element of KP's success. The organization operates on a technology platform matched by few others in health care anywhere in the world—in size, scope, and capability. In the United States, barely more than half the number of doctors use an electronic health record (EHR); at KP, EHR use is at 100 percent. Dr. Jed Weissberg, senior vice president for hospitals, quality, and care delivery excellence at KP, who is also a practicing physician, considers widespread physician and patient adoption of secured e-mail messaging to be foundational. The ability of doctors and patients to communicate directly and rapidly is an immensely powerful clinical tool.

"We have millions of e-mail messages going back and forth every year," says Weissberg. "It is an intrinsic part of medical care now when it wasn't 10 years ago. It is now spread throughout the organization. I think that is a profound transforming mode of communication between the care delivery system and patients."

Why is this so critical to clinical quality? Why is it—in the words of KP CEO George Halvorson—such "a huge breakthrough"? Because when patients are connected with ready access to their care teams as well as to the full array of their own health information and records, they are more engaged in their care and thus in their health. They are less likely to get lost in the netherworld of "between visit" care.

KP technology does much more than enable close communication between patients and care teams and empowering patients to become more engaged in their care. It also aggregates and analyzes massive quantities of data from tens of millions of patient encounters throughout the country. In addition to this technology, KP clinicians also have access to one of the most important and useful electronic libraries in the world—the Kaiser Permanente Clinical Library, a compendium of research-based guidelines, evidence products and reference materials.

## Innovations from the KP Care Management Institute

The library finds its home within the KP Care Management Institute (CMI), a modest-sized operation within KP whose impact on research, evidence-based guidelines, and ultimately delivery of care at the front lines is immeasurable. CMI is a national R&D center that tests and spreads new clinical approaches and harnesses technology to spread evidence-based care as it strives to foster care coordination and patient centeredness.

In the initial portion of this chapter we focus largely on the work of CMI, particularly as it relates to three of the central clinical challenges of our time—heart disease, obesity, and cancer care. In an article titled "The Care Management Instutute: Making the Right Thing Easier to Do" (2005) Dr. Paul Wallace, then executive director of CMI, wrote that

> The creation of rigorous, evidence-based clinical content is the foundation of CMI's work. Interregional workgroups consisting of clinical experts from medicine, pharmacy, and nursing, evidence-based methodologists, and CMI care management consultants have created clinical practice guidelines for a core set of conditions and health care issues: asthma, coronary artery disease, chronic pain, cancer, depression, diabetes, elder care, heart failure, and self-care and shared decision making. These guidelines have been

approved on a national level by the National Guideline Directors, representing all regions, and are revised at least every two years.

CMI is an expert convener, drawing together experienced professionals with expertise in many clinical areas as well as in outcomes measurement, evidence-based guidelines development, and epidemiology. CMI is led by co-directors—Dr. Scott Young, a practicing physician who is also senior medical director, and Alide Chase, senior vice president, quality and safety. A key to CMI's success is that it's relatively modest-sized central staff of 52 professionals is constantly reaching out to solicit and embrace ideas and suggestions from throughout the KP system. "It's not that CMI is doing all the thinking themselves," says Weissberg. "What makes CMI really successful is the ability to harness the greater power of thinking and experience from throughout KP. CMI is the focus and nexus for learning and operational improvement. We have interaction between thought leaders and practice leaders to try things in an operational setting until we find something that works."

## Breakthrough for Complex Cardiovascular Patients

The pathway to achieving the Triple Aim travels directly through the epidemic of heart disease and other chronic conditions that challenge tens of millions of Americans and account for a staggering percentage of health care costs. Treating high-risk patients with diabetes, heart disease, or both—including those who have experienced a prior heart attack—is exceptionally challenging. These patients not only have a markedly higher probability of suffering a stroke or heart attack than patients without these prior conditions, but they also represent a formidable challenge to the nation's clinical and financial resources.

"In many ways, our journey around heart disease has been job one at CMI," says Dr. Scott Young. "Ten or fifteen years ago that was *the* disease. We worked at understanding where people were doing this well and how we could get to guidelines. CMI was first to bring in population-based performance measures around heart disease. We could say, 'This group of patients is doing better than this group. What are the clinicians doing differently?'"

After much study, CMI created evidence-based guidelines for KP clinical teams to use at the point of care. KP began a program in 2003 to help high-risk heart patients avoid serious complications of cardiovascular disease. This was known as the A-L-L Initiative (Aspirin-Lipid-lowering therapy-Lisinopril). KP researchers prescribed a drug combination of both a statin (lovastatin 40 mg) and a blood pressure medication (lisinopril 20 mg). Many patients also took a low-dose aspirin.

KP used the Archimedes simulation model, says Weissberg, which "showed that putting people with cardiovascular risk above a certain level—putting them on aspirin, medicine from the ACE inhibitor group, and a statin would dramatically lower their risk of heart attack or stroke. That made us want to take a much more proactive stance."

Clinicians knew that for patients with diabetes or heart disease these three drugs, which are quite inexpensive in the overall scheme of things, reduced the risk of future heart attacks and strokes. Clinicians theorized that widespread use of the three drugs together in high-risk patients could have a major impact on health and mortality. The challenge was to identify those patients and to get them on the medications—and here is where KP's size, reach, and technological sophistication played a pivotal role in helping clinicians identify high-risk patients.

In 2007, after two years of administering the medicines to a target audience, CMI conducted a research project studying nearly 70,000 patients. An internal KP report indicated that "while previous research and clinical trials have shown that" the A-L-L medications "individually reduce heart attacks and strokes, this is the first study to evaluate whether a consistent process could be developed to deliver the combined drugs to large numbers of people with diabetes and/or heart disease in realistic settings across a health care delivery system. It is also the first study to evaluate how dramatically this program would affect clinical outcomes and hospitalization rates for heart attack and stroke."

The results of the study were a triumph for the A-L-L approach. CMI researchers reported in an *American Journal of Managed Care* article (Dudl, Wang, Wong, & Bellows, 2009) that patients in the study reduced their risk of stroke or heart attack by up to 80 percent and that even patients who only took the drugs part of the time significantly reduced their risk. Dr. R. James Dudl, who led the study and serves as diabetes clinical leader at CMI, told Reuters, "Even in people who took it less than half the time, they got over a 60 percent drop in heart attacks and strokes. Those who took it more than half the time, they got more like an 80 percent drop."

The CMI study found that this approach improves the quality of individual care, has a huge impact on populations of at-risk patients, and drives down the cost of care (Steenhuysen, 2009).

"We made the right thing to do the easy thing to do with cardiovascular disease with guidelines and tools at the point of care," says Dr. Young. CMI's work in cardiovascular disease has enabled KP to identify the best evidence and to place guidelines and tools at the point of care that are easily used by clinical care teams.

## Going Upstream to Work on Obesity

KP's sustained effort on improving care for people with heart disease and diabetes inevitably led the organization to focus on obesity. Working to reduce obesity demands not only intensive effort with patients and care teams, but also requires working with others outside the traditional boundaries of the health care system. Most determinants of health, in fact, reside far outside the clinical realm in the everyday lives and habits of patients—they occur "upstream" from the ailments and conditions patients present with at a clinic visit.

Hence, to tackle obesity, KP joined the Convergence Partnership, a coalition of health care leaders from a number of other organizations, including The California Endowment, Kresge Foundation, Robert Wood Johnson Foundation, W.K. Kellogg Foundation, and Nemours, among others. In a May 2010 letter to US Department of Health and Human Services Secretary Kathleen Sebelius, these leaders, including KP senior vice president Raymond J. Baxter, PhD, wrote (Convergence Partnership, 2010):

> While access to health care is critical, a large and growing body of research shows that health status is influenced far more by the environments in which we live, work, learn, and play. These

environments have a profound impact on individuals' diet, physical activity, and safety. . . Research shows that health problems are linked to conditions in communities. The neighborhoods where we live—whether we have access to healthy food, safe places to walk and play, good housing, steady jobs, connections with neighbors, friends, and community institutions—influence our health status. Therefore, if we are to improve health and prevent disease and injury, we must attend to the environments surrounding people.

Says Dr. Young: "Obesity is hard. It is an overwhelming causative and contributing factor to the vast majority of chronic and ongoing life-threatening conditions we see, [including] cancer. At our annual meeting one of the cancer physicians said to me, 'If you can't fix the obesity problem in our population, we can't fix the cancer problem.' Fifty to 75 percent of cancers are caused by lifestyle (e.g., smoking, being sedentary). Women who are obese and had breast cancer are at increased risk for recurrence. You can't chemotherapy your way out of the cancer problem. You have to prevent it."

There is no easy fix for obesity. "You cannot solve it in the exam room alone," says Young. "It involves communities, schools—a whole different set of partners than we have [had] in the past. We're starting to put together communities of interest very different than the ones we've had. [For] childhood obesity, you ask: How can I influence schools? How can I influence choices at home?"

While finding ways to reduce obesity is immensely challenging, complex work, it is potentially transformative for it goes right to the heart of the Triple Aim. An important step forward has been the decision at some KP hospitals and clinics to include exercise as a "vital sign." "Several of our facilities are making it a standard protocol," says Young. "You check in for your appointment and we take your blood pressure, pulse, height, weight, and the medical assistant asks how much physical exercise you get on a typical day. She enters that into the record and it will prompt the clinician to have a discussion around it." That conversation will focus on getting the patient to do *something*; walk, for example.

KP is going upstream and engaging with communities in many ways including community health initiatives such as

Healthy Eating Active Living, a grass roots initiative promoting exactly what the title suggests. "Wouldn't it be great if you never had to go on a blood pressure pill or if we could help you not have to see a cardiologist?" Young asks. "Yes, we want to prevent someone with high blood pressure from having a heart attack, but we would rather prevent you from having high blood pressure in the first place. One is health care and one is health."

Weissberg asks: "How can clinical care extend out into the community? We partner with our community benefits department to promote the concept of total health with schools in our service areas through school nurses, changes in the cafeteria [food choices], and working to make sure the areas around schools are safe places to walk and play and exercise."

A new initiative launched in 2012 involves KP partnering with HBO, the Institute of Medicine, the Centers for Disease Control and Prevention, the National Institutes of Health, and the Michael and Susan Dell Foundation to create a public campaign targeting obesity (http://theweightofthenation.hbo.com/#). The campaign includes a series of documentary films, a community-based outreach campaign, as well as a social media initiative to combat obesity through awareness and education. The ultimate goal is to put on display strategies that work in controlling weight and getting people to act upon those strategies.

## Standardized, Effective, Measurable Cancer Care

CMI works to support regional initiatives on cancer care in much the same way it works on heart disease and other issues, says Young. "We want to be patient-focused, systematic, and evidence-based," he says. "We want to be able to measure our outcomes and capitalize on people in the KP system who did better." CMI works with clinicians throughout the national KP system to identify breakthrough strategies for cancer care. By drawing on the collective wisdom and experience these clinicians have with treating millions of cancer patients through the years, CMI is in a powerful position to create better standard practices and spread them throughout KP.

After a good deal of success in their work with heart disease, regional clinical leaders decided to take a broad look at cancer care, and once again they engaged the CMI team. "What does complete cancer care look like?" Young asks. "What do the paths look like? What are the metrics, the evidence? And what has come into focus is that, as opposed to cardiac conditions, in cancer there are many, many, many more conditions. There is lung cancer and thyroid cancer, and there are different causes and different treatments and they impact different people in different ways."

Thus, he says, in some respects the challenge with cancer care is even greater than with heart disease. CMI research revealed that throughout KP there were four thousand different protocols for delivery of cancer drugs to patients. According to an internal KP report, CMI found that "prior to 2008, chemotherapy ordering and administration across KP was predominately paper-based. Standardization of chemotherapy regimens was rare and driven by prescriber preference."

"We took a tour of the country looking for metrics indicating great cancer care and it was all different," says Young. "We came back and said, 'We have to get common protocols and metrics out there.'"

Variation meant the quality and effectiveness of chemotherapy protocols was unpredictable. In an area as complex as cancer care, how was anyone to know whether the approach used by Dr. Smith was as effective as the approach used by Dr. Jones—on similar patients with comparable cancers?

CMI provided support for KP oncologists as they identified the most effective chemotherapy treatments and subsequently defined fourteen hundred standard chemotherapy approaches which were then integrated into the KP HealthConnect® electronic system. The result was that clinicians could identify the best evidence-based drug treatment for any type of cancer right there on the electronic health record at the point of care.

This breakthrough resulted in much more consistent, standardized delivery of effective care to cancer patients. Technology played a pivotal role in this work. The KP team introduced a new aspect of the electronic record—called the KP HealthConnect Beacon® Oncology Module—that enables clinicians to identify the best evidence-based practice for cancer patients much more rapidly and effectively than before. An Institute of Medicine (IOM) member spotlight article reported that the Beacon Module "supports high-quality, evidence-based, safe care for all KP oncology patients across four regions." The article also noted that a KP team "decreased the number of chemotherapy protocols. . . for orders, replications, fluids, rates of administration, and nursing notes—through an evidence review and consensus development process that vetted oncologists, pharmacists, and nurses from each region. . . In order to quickly modify KP's standardized order sets as evidence evolves and emerges, oncologists also have organized themselves into groups to review the latest evidence emerging from cancer journals and important conferences."

The IOM article noted some results from the Beacon Module at KP:

- 84 percent or higher adherence to evidence-based templates across regions
- 9 percent reduction in adverse events at the San Jose Medical Center (pilot site)
- 18 percent reduction in oncology nursing overtime (based on evaluation of 8 Northern California facilities)
- 48-hour response time for notification of leukemia drug (Mylotarg) recall, cessation of recalled drug use, and arrangement of alternative therapies in all Beacon live regions
- Increased capability to manage pharmacy and biotechnology resources and respond quickly to new knowledge about treatments or drug efficacy
- Rapid implementation of new protocols in response to changes in the evidence base (e.g., use of Avastin following changes in reported efficacy data from the American Society of Clinical Oncology)
- Growing database for treatment outcomes research

The KP team succeeded in reducing the number of protocols for administering chemotherapy from fourteen hundred to seven hundred standard approaches, thus substantially minimizing treatment variations that were once based on the personal preference of a particular doctor. This standardization has enabled KP to measure the effectiveness of various protocols much more effectively.

"The Beacon Oncology Module is a component on our electronic record that essentially lets our oncologists have one standard order set for adult tumors for chemotherapy," says Young. "This is instead of all those cocktails for different cancers. Beacon has real promise to revolutionize adult cancer treatment." And this decision is partly the result of the work supported by CMI in conjunction with oncologists and other clinicians throughout the country to identify and agree on best practices.

Of course, the pace of cancer research these days is fast and very little in the treatment of the disease is static—at least not for long. So, what happens when new evidence suggests the need for new treatments? "We can respond very, very quickly in our oncologist practices," says Weissberg. The CMI team consults with an existing panel of cancer experts and the judgment is made based on the new evidence whether or not to change the care protocol. In cases where change is required, the new protocol is rapidly installed in the electronic system and information about it is spread to all cancer care providers at KP. As powerful as this research is in providing clinicians with the best information on treatments, KP has also focused on improving the quality, safety, and efficiency of care by focusing on the frontline experiences of patients and staff.

## Video Ethnography: A Powerful CMI Tool for Spread

Another key improvement that hails from CMI's work is the use of video ethnography, which has become an effective tool for innovation and spread at KP. Estee Neuwirth, PhD, director of field studies at CMI, leads the work in video ethnography. She explains that *ethnography*, or field work, "is a qualitative method that involves interviews and observation to understand, interpret, and describe experience, systems, organizations, and cultures," and thus *video ethnography* is "the rapid, applied use of ethnographic methods using video to capture observation and interviews in order to analyze and then share key findings. . . with quality improvement teams, leaders, and others across an organization or institution."

The technique is simple. A particular process—for example, medication administration on a hospital unit—is chosen as the focus. Using a small, handheld video camera, one team member spends a couple of days videotaping nurses and other clinicians interacting with patients around medication administration. In total, there might be as much as fifteen hours of video after two days of filming. Several members of the video ethnography team review and edit the video down to a three- to five-minute sample that is intended to show the key elements of the process (e.g., medication administration).

"It's a challenge in health care. . . to identify gaps and opportunities to improve and build will for change and real understanding of the patient," says Neuwirth. "Video ethnography is a tool for that purpose."

When Neuwirth does videotaping, she asks patients and staff members simple questions and films their answers: What is the experience like? How could it be better? What do you want and need to help you get better? What do you want and need to do your job more effectively? To make your work more rewarding?

A related technique, and one that predates video ethnography, is *shadowing*, in which a staff member follows other team members or patients around to observe and record in writing the precise nature of their experience. But Neuwirth finds video ethnography to be even more effective than shadowing. "Video changes the whole nature of it," she says. "With video, everyone sees when things are and are not working."

Neuwirth describes video ethnography as a tool "that allows us all to see care delivery even more clearly from the eyes of our patients. The advantage of using video ethnography is that we can share these patient stories and important themes from interviews with patients and staff widely across the organization, and this tool is proving to be a powerful catalyst for spread and improvement."

Neuwirth and her colleagues have used video ethnography in a wide variety of areas, ranging from readmissions and diabetes care to surgical pre-op and medication management. There have been many moments when the resulting videotape has presented a defining moment for caregivers. The CMI project on improving transitions from the hospital to home is a good example. These transitions, of course, are fraught with opportunities for mistakes. Typically, a patient—often frail and perhaps elderly— is given crucial instructions before being sent home. If these instructions are effective, why have hospital readmissions been increasing in the United States?

Dr. Weissberg characterizes video ethnography as "the single most dramatic change in the way we think about care that I have seen in 28 years." He says when KP was doing the initial work on transitions of care from hospital to home, the CMI team watched a video as the patient, in her hospital room, was spoken to "by a succession of well-intentioned people coming in and talking about medications, dietary issues, explaining how to get in touch with physicians—one person after another coming into the room and giving her instructions."

The patient was also videotaped about her experience, saying "all of that was well and good, but I just want to get out of here!"

As a result of such findings using video ethnography, KP developed a bundle of interventions for transitioning patients from the hospital to home (Figure 7.1) that includes conducting more extensive post-hospitalization follow-ups and giving discharged patients an easy way to reach a caregiver—a designated phone number that patients can use to get timely answers to their clinical questions.

**Figure 7.1. Elements in the New Transition Bundle Spreading Across KP**

| What does the patient and family need? | Transition bundle |
| --- | --- |
| I will have what I need when I return home. | ▪ Risk Stratification with tailored care <br> ▪ Standardized RN/CC Needs Assessment |
| I know when I should call and what number to use when I need help. | ▪ Specialized phone number on DC Instructions |
| My regular doctor will know what happened to me in the hospital. | ▪ Standardized Same Day Discharge Summary |
| I understand my medications, how to take them, and why I need them. | ▪ Pharmacist reviewing medications in hospital <br> ▪ PharmD phone call (high risk) |
| I know someone will check on me when I am home. | ▪ MD appointments made in hospital within 5 (high risk) to 10 days <br> ▪ RN follow up call within 48 hours <br> ▪ RN case mgmt 30 days (high risk) |

"We reframed how we think about our interventions," Neuwirth says, "so that all interventions are linked to what patients want and need. From that ethnographic work we learned that emotional goals of patients and caregivers affected the amount of information they absorbed on discharge day. We also found that same-day discharge teaching can be ineffective because patients can be anxious about leaving the hospital or staff members may feel rushed. Emotion can interfere with cognition, and transferring information shortly before hospital discharge may overlook learning readiness, a fundamental principle of patient education."

Neuwirth sees video ethnography as a simple, inexpensive tool that anyone in health care can use to build will for change, to generate new ideas for improvement, and to determine whether staff members are executing improvements reliably. "It brings the voice of patient into the room and changes the whole conversation," says Neuwirth. "When we interview a range of patients, we see patterns and themes."

Since 2010, she has trained more than twenty ten-member unit-based teams in the technique, and all of them have applied video ethnography successfully in improvement projects.

## KP Innovation Consultancy

The Care Management Institute is not the only place within KP that has a crucial innovation and improvement role. In fact, that assignment is marbled throughout the organization. KP's Innovation Consultancy, for example, is one of those entities. The Innovation Consultancy is an internal design group founded in 2003 that works on innovation and on spreading new methods throughout Kaiser Permanente. Chris McCarthy, an innovation team member, describes the consultancy as "an evidence-based, human-centered design group"—a unique combination of approaches. It blends what McCarthy calls a "traditional ideation phase—synthesis, brainstorming, prototyping, etc.—and then we tag on the science of improvement," which includes field-testing and the establishment of outcome and process metrics. "We go from nothing all the way to testing ideas and proving that these ideas will provide value," he says. "We call that innovation only if we *know* it provides value. Up until then, it is just a concept or an idea."

In 2007, Christi Zuber, head of the Innovation Consultancy, and McCarthy asked some nurses at KP what was wrong with medication administration. The initial response from the nurses seemed to end the discussion. "There is nothing wrong," the nurses said. "We work hard and get it done."

Zuber and McCarthy wanted to dig deeper. Experience taught them that frequently there was a disconnect between what people in health care were thinking and what they were feeling. McCarthy sat down with a number of nurses and, in an organization with billions of dollars worth of technology, he handed them crayons, colored markers, and blank sheets of paper. He asked them to reflect on what came to mind when they focused on the idea of *medication administration*, then to visualize it and draw whatever image came to mind on a sheet of paper.

In about fifteen minutes he had an answer that was the polar opposite of what the nurses had told him verbally (Figures 7.2

**Figure 7.2. Nurse's Visualization of Medication Administration: 1**

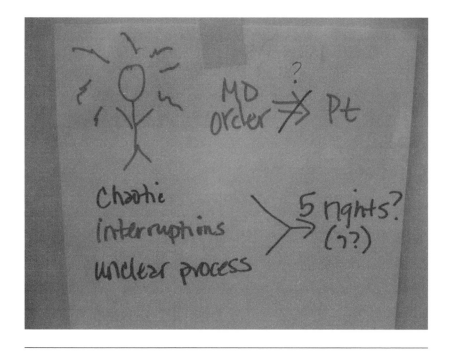

**Figure 7.3. Nurse's Visualization of Medication Administration: 2**

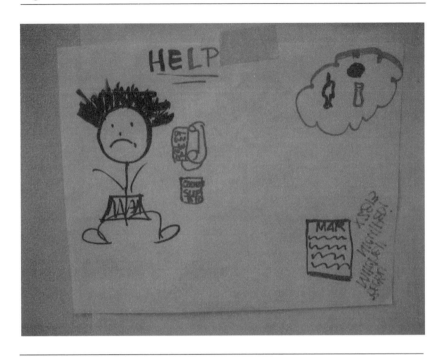

and 7.3 display two of the nurses' drawings). McCarthy says, "In the drawings nurses looked upset, sad, frustrated, and frazzled." And when McCarthy and Zuber pursued the content of these drawings, the nurses then told them that medication administration was chaotic, unsettling, sometimes unclear, and packed with interruptions.

"We did several studies and we documented the interrupts and they were big," says McCarthy. "I documented one [medication administration] that had 17 interrupts! Now that was extreme. The average was about one interruption per administration and even that is really high. Imagine *every* medication administration being interrupted."

After seeing the nurses' drawings and digging deeper to understand their concerns and frustrations with medication administration, McCarthy pulled together a pilot group of nurses, doctors, pharmacists, and patients to visit companies in a number of different industries. He wanted the group to witness firsthand how companies outside of health care worked relentlessly to improve safety over years or even decades. The group visited a flight school, a Lexus car dealership, and a Safeway supermarket, and then spent two days working together on ideas to improve medication safety within KP. They convened at the Kaiser Permanente Sidney R. Garfield Health Care Innovation Center, a simulation space where KP teams tested a wide variety of ideas before attempting to implement them within the system. (The Garfield Center may be unique in all of health care—we'll talk more about it later in this chapter.)

During their two days at Garfield, the team members were infused with energy. There was a palpable sense that working together they could make an impact—maybe a big impact—on medication safety. The team talked about virtually every aspect of medication administration. In all, about four hundred ideas were proposed and forty of them were intriguing enough to inspire the team to construct quick prototypes, using such simple materials as paper, cardboard, markers, and tape. From these forty prototypes, the team then selected a total of fifteen for further study and possible development.

One of the quick mock-ups was a large bib with a pink sign that said "LEAVE ME ALONE" that a nurse would wear when doing medication administration. When the team at the Garfield Center saw it everyone laughed. McCarthy and his colleagues loved this idea—not the *leave me alone* part but the underlying idea of what they quickly dubbed *no-interruption wear,* a garment that would signal to all that the nurse was in the process of delivering medication and must not be interrupted.

The idea was compelling. It was given the formal name of KP MedRite, the KP methodology for delivering medication to patients in the safest possible manner. Over a ten-month period, the idea was prototyped, revised repeatedly, and piloted. In the Sacramento pilot site, the team bought a $10 safety vest at Home Depot and tried it out as their no-interruption wear prototype. The nurses liked the idea of a garment sending the no-interruption signal, but they did not like the large, clumsy vest. The next iteration of the idea was a wide sash but, again, it was too cumbersome. Nurses wanted something slimmer that they could fold up and carry in a pocket. And that is precisely what they got.

## The Failure Path to Spread and Improvement

"A lot of our projects end up successful because we go through rapid failures early on, and I think the sash is a really good example of that—where at first the idea sounds really good, but when you try it out in practice, the feedback might be negative," says McCarthy. "But generally folks are able to articulate what would make an idea work and, as long as they can continue to articulate what would make it work, that gives you the momentum to keep moving forward. We kept taking the idea [of no-interruption wear] and iterated it over and over again to a successful conclusion."

An important addition to the KP MedRite process included defining a *sacred zone*, an area clearly marked on the unit floor. When a nurse is in that zone working on dispensing medications, no other caregiver is permitted to enter that space. It is an enhancement to the no-interruption theme of KP MedRite that gives the nurse the space needed to focus completely on the medication task at hand.

The question during field-testing is simple: Do the people who will be applying the idea like the idea? If they like the idea, then McCarthy and colleagues start thinking about how to test it in pilot sites, a process that may take anywhere from three months to a year or more. KP prefers to conduct pilot tests in a minimum of two locations and in at least two different KP regions, for a total of four pilots.

When the idea works in multiple locations then it is deemed ready for spread, and spread begins with the creation of a *change package* that explains the new process and provides a variety of tools for local teams to use toward implementation. Each change package is prepared in three versions, one for each of three organizational levels: frontline staff, implementation manager, and leader. Change packages feature excellent graphics and clear, straightforward writing that tends to grab the attention of the target audience.

The change packages include a good deal of material posted on an internal Web site that can be used in various locations to promote spread. All the tools developed to spread or communicate about the innovation can be downloaded by staff.

Posters and other material, for example, can be downloaded and printed so each hospital doesn't have to re-create the communication materials. Change packages may also include videos that show what a new innovation should look like—how it should work and flow.

When an innovation is being spread, the quality of the change package is important, and the KP project teams work hard to make their change packages among the best. In fact, some years back IHI leaders recognized KP's change packages as a best practice. The change packages have been made available for other organizations to download and use, and numerous health organizations in North America beyond KP have adopted the KP MedRite practices (http://xnet.kp.org/innovationconsultancy/kpmedrite.html).

Beyond the change package features already described, there are two additional important elements. A package needs to describe the failure path and establish minimum specifications. Successful spread, says McCarthy, often depends on frontline workers knowing the details of what did not work and seeing the sequence of change during the design and testing process. "When I walk people down the failure path, somehow that enables them to accept the final idea without having to add feedback to it. . . As I am walking the failure path for you, you are visualizing yourself participating in the failure and. . . the suggestion of how to make it better."

## The Power of Minimum Specifications

Weighing down innovations with multiple specifications hinders spread. "A big pitfall we find is organizations saying, 'This is the answer—these three things, and this is how you have to do it in order to get it right,'" says McCarthy. "Instead, we have a minimum specification that we use, and this comes from thinking that your organization is human rather than robotic—rather than this computer that you can just program." In KP MedRite the minimum specifications focus on three components: a tool, a space, and a process. The tool is the no-interruption sash. The space is the sacred space. And the process for the nurse is as follows:

- Enter the medication room wearing the no-interruption sash.
- Check the five rights of medication administration: right medication, right time, right patient, right dose, right route.
- Proceed to the patient's room, sanitize hands, and inform the patient that it is time for medication.
- Explain clearly to the patient what medication is being administered and why it is being used.
- Use the barcoding scanner to document medication administration in the electronic medical record.
- Sanitize hands again, remove sash, and leave patient's room.

In the KP Northwest region the nurses discussed alternative ideas and came up with a medication tray that was the exact same, highly visible, bright green color as the sash. "Who cares if [the tool] is a sash or if it is a medication tray?" says McCarthy. "We care that it is *no interruption.*"

Part of the idea of providing minimum specifications is that this enables workers to adapt and change the idea for their local context. "We really believe in allowing individual units to have some of their DNA put into the innovation, and that increases the stickiness, the sustainability," says McCarthy. "When they do that, their thinking is, 'I put my time and energy myself into it; I want this thing to work.'"

## KP MedRite Results

With KP MedRite, interruptions were reduced from an average of 1 for every medication delivery to 0.2 per delivery. Prior to KP MedRite, 68 percent of nurses said that the medication administration process was clear, safe, and easy. After KP MedRite was in place that number increased to over 90 percent. Significantly, the new system improved the likelihood that the basic five steps of medication administration would be covered, improving compliance from 33 percent before KP MedRite to nearly 80 percent afterward.

## Building a Performance System Throughout KP

Kaiser Permanente chairman and CEO George Halvorson loved the work done by the Care Management Institute, as well as the work the Innovation Consultancy had done with KP MedRite. Halvorson knew as well as anyone how innovative Kaiser Permanente had been through the years. He clearly understood that innovation was part of the nature of the place. But Halvorson wanted more. He wanted an improvement capacity *everywhere*—in every KP hospital, clinic, and physician's office. He wanted more than a culture of innovation. He wanted the capacity to innovate, improve, and spread woven throughout the fabric of the organization.

In November 2007, Halvorson sat down with a number of executives, including Alide Chase. Chase recalls, "He said, 'I would like you to build a performance improvement system in the organization.'" Halvorson wanted an organizational approach to performance improvement; to build capacity and skill to improve. He wanted it to draw on the best improvement practices in health care, but he also wanted it to fit comfortably within KP. And he wanted to start the work on KP's front lines of care.

It was a challenging time at KP. The organization was then in the process of finishing the implementation of its electronic health record, Kaiser Permanente HealthConnect. "As we finished execution of KP HealthConnect, we were going to need to leverage this tremendous IT investment we made," says Chase, "by having the skill and people for performance improvement. We needed to marry the IT wizardry with skill-building capacity for staff." It was Chase's responsibility to lead the effort to turn Halvorson's vision into reality. There were many questions: What would the performance model look like? What components would be included? What skills and capabilities would have to be built into the organization?

From the start, Chase and other improvement experts— including Chris McCarthy and Lisa Schilling, vice president of healthcare performance improvement at KP—knew what they did *not* want: They did not want a project-based improvement process. Many organizations in health care tended in that direction. With a project approach, these organizations would select an issue—say, medication safety—and build a team of clinicians to focus on that topic and oftentimes make very good progress. Some time later the same organization might be facing a challenge around wait times and might build a team to do a project around that. "The teams become subject matter experts," says McCarthy. "The thing that is missing is that there is no transfer of knowledge" about *how to innovate and improve*. "All the skills and techniques the first team worked hard to learn—learning how to innovate—none of that is transferred to the next team."

George Halvorson wanted to do something much more ambitious—to embed continuous quality improvement knowledge within the organization's infrastructure so that experts in innovation and improvement techniques could join teams of subject matter experts and bring powerful improvement knowledge and experience to the table.

Chase and Schilling initiated a series of visits in 2007 to a variety of different health care organizations that were among the best in the world, including Intermountain Healthcare, where Dr. Brent James had developed a renowned improvement curriculum many years earlier. They liked the improvement approaches undertaken by other places as well, including Cincinnati Children's Hospital Medical Center, Ascension Health, SSM Healthcare, and Jönköping County in Sweden. These organizations had been working diligently on internal improvement and spread for years. All had significant investments of time and talent within their own systems. At IHI, Improvement Advisors helped connect the KP performance improvement team with these organizations.

"We were going to different places to learn how the best organizations ahead of us were already doing things," says Chase. "IHI had relationships with all of these places and they knew who was way downstream."

Schilling returned from visiting other sites and wrote a paper analyzing where KP stood and recommending a path forward. She observed that KP "does not have consistent structures and processes for sustained performance improvement to enable world-class performance across all levels of the organization." Schilling says that studying the work at various organizations resulted in the KP team identifying "six essential capabilities to creating high-performing organizations":

1. Leadership and the ability of leaders to identify the "vital few breakthrough opportunities";
2. A systems approach;
3. Measurement capability at all levels;
4. The culture of a learning organization (with an "infrastructure to harvest best practices for sharing and learning to create potential for spreading practices with the greatest impact");
5. Team engagement from the bottom up; and
6. A strong internal capability to improve.

"We wanted to get the improvement skill level as close to the front lines as possible," says Chase. "We didn't want to build a national improvement center."

## Unit-Based Teams

"We wanted a majority of the skill building to occur as close to the facility where clinical care was provided as possible," says Chase, and that meant engaging with what KP calls *unit-based teams* (UBTs), defined as "all the participants in a natural work unit or department, including supervisors, union stewards and staff members, physicians, nurses, dentists, and managers." These teams were a product of an agreement negotiated in 2005 between KP and its unions as a way to improve care for patients, while providing the best possible work environment for employees.

John August, executive director of the Coalition of Kaiser Permanente Unions, makes the case that "the foundation of the partnership" between KP and its unions is performance improvement. August notes that the National Agreement of KP and its unions "commits us to changing the organizational culture to support whole system improvement. . . The goal is to achieve continuous improvement on many measures of performance improvement all at once, rather than focus on improvement initiative by initiative or project by project" (August, 2010).

**Figure 7.4. The KP Value Compass**

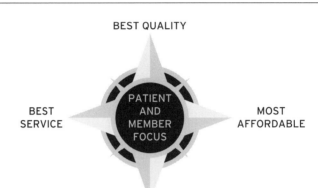

This alignment of labor and management around quality and improvement has provided KP with great flexibility and freedom at both local and regional levels in the pursuit of improvement. This is foundational to innovation. In health care, change and improvement are nearly always challenging and often painful. If management-labor conflict is added to that challenge, then change and improvement become exponentially more difficult. The KP arrangement helps to alleviate some of this strife. More specifically, the UBTs are guided by the KP Value Compass (Figure 7.4) which puts a patient and member focus at the center of performance improvement, and indeed at the center of all that staff do at Kaiser Permanente.

## From Project to Portfolio

In the winter of 2008, Chase, Schilling, and other performance improvement team members launched an Improvement Institute for executives and Improvement Advisor (IA) trainees. This program was to be the nucleus of the improvement capacity that CEO George Halvorson aspired to spread throughout KP. The purpose of the program was to train large numbers of KP employees how to serve as skilled guides in helping KP teams improve any internal process. While they would not be subject matter experts in all areas, they would possess operational expertise in the art and science of improvement.

From the start, the IA trainees were taught to think in terms of an improvement *portfolio* rather than individual improvement projects. The concept of IAs having a portfolio of projects is fundamental to the success of the KP approach, and Chase stresses the difference between project management and portfolio management. In a project approach a team might focus, for example, just on applying the ventilator-acquired pneumonia (VAP) bundle effectively. With a portfolio approach, however, IAs align each implementation with the overall strategic plan of the organization. For example, if a hospital's goal is to reduce infections, then the IA will look at the challenge broadly. The work will involve implementing the VAP bundle effectively, of course. But that activity alone may not reduce overall infections in the hospital, or it may have only a marginal impact. Thus the IA also will get involved with work related to preventing infections from central lines, improving staff hand washing compliance, and improving the sanitary conditions of rooms, bed linens, equipment, and more. When an IA makes "the jump from a project to a portfolio, the senior leader says to go for a. . . *Big Dot*," says Chase. A Big Dot is a whole-system measure (such as "reduce our inpatient mortality rate by 20 percent within two years") that can be used to rate performance and effectiveness and to align incentives (Pugh and Reinertsen, 2007). Then, says Chase, the IA has "to take on several projects in several units that will form a portfolio, and as the skill of the IA increases so does their ability to deal with many teams. The ability to see the whole is what happens when you move to a portfolio [perspective]."

Faculty for the Improvement Advisor program, drawn largely from outside KP, included Dr. Uma Kotagal from Cincinnati Children's Hospital Medical Center, Lynn Maher from the National Health Service innovation consultancy in England, and a number of individuals from IHI, including Robert Lloyd. IHI president and CEO Maureen Bisognano, co-author of this book, taught participants about the leader's role in improvement.

## The Rapid Improvement Model and Other Tools

The instructors' work is to "put tools in the IA trainees' toolkit," says Chase. For example, IAs learn some basic ethnography, flow-mapping, and cost analysis skills. During the coursework, instructors and mentors are on the floor, circulating among, advising, and assisting the IA trainees.

"We teach things like how to set a goal, how to run a test, and [employ] statistics so you can see improvement over time," says Schilling. "How do you look at a process and standardize and simplify the process so it is easy to do the right thing? Where do you get started? How do you pilot locally? How do you move to the next site? How do you optimize, and how do you monitor and oversee improvement?"

An essential element of succeeding under this model for improvement is making sure that all Improvement Advisors have an excellent working knowledge of rapid-cycle testing—PDSA (Plan-Do-Study-Act) tests that can be conducted, analyzed, and measured very quickly. "Everyone has to have this rapid improvement model knowledge," says Chase. "The IAs in training learn how to figure out over the next ninety days how to reliably execute on a bundle of practices, and try small PDSAs and keep measuring to see how reliably we execute the bundle."

"What knowledge does everyone need to have?" Schilling asks. "We believe that everybody needs to know basically the Model for Improvement and rapid tests of change." This core of the IA training was the approach enunciated in a book that has become a classic in the literature of improvement science, *The Improvement Guide: A Practical Approach to Enhancing Organizational Performance* (Langley, Moen, Nolan, Nolan, Norman, and Provost, 2009).

- **Setting goals.** What is our overall goal with this initiative? What are we trying to accomplish? Instructors show students that effective improvement requires precise definition of what is to be accomplished, with measurable, time-specific goals.
- **Identifying measurements.** What exactly will we measure to determine whether we are making progress?
- **Identifying changes.** What specific changes can we make that will lead to improvement? As the teams at KP like to say

(paraphrasing Don Berwick), "all improvement requires making changes, but not all changes result in improvement." It is essential to focus on changes that have the potential to effect real change.

- **Testing outcomes.** Finally, students are taught how to apply the basic PDSA cycle to test change. With effective use of PDSA, the IAs and their teams will plan together, do the work together, study the results together, and act to adjust or implement.

By the end of 2011—less than three years after the start of the Improvement Institute and the IA training program—KP completed three waves of training that put a total of more than one thousand Improvement Advisors into the ranks, and KP was well into the fourth wave with a total of three hundred additional IAs in training. In addition, KP has developed an even more rigorous curriculum for a new category of more advanced and highly trained Improvement Advisors.

Once IAs graduate from the training program, having completed their first ninety-day improvement cycle, they quickly move to the next project in their portfolio. "We want the improvement capability immediately applied to the next area of priority in the strategic plan," says Chase. "So the IA in a given area is working on something while the next IA is in training right on their heels." By the end of 2011, KP's unit-based teams, led by the internally trained Improvement Advisors, completed more than ten thousand patient-centered performance improvement projects.

The collective impact of thousands of projects throughout KP is difficult to overestimate. Constant improvement and the internal KP ability to accelerate that improvement by training more and more Improvement Advisors impacts specific areas throughout KP, of course, but it also serves as an engine that helps drive the "big dots" on patient satisfaction, clinical outcomes, and costs.

## Creating Nurse Knowledge Exchange

It is difficult to overstate the importance of transitions in care in any setting, but especially in an acute care hospital. For nurses, shift changes constitute a never-ending relay race. Throughout the field of health care, in facilities large and small, urban and rural, the shift change is a crucial moment that presents significant challenges. But within this pivotal period of time also lies the opportunity to create systems and procedures that provide better, safer care for patients. A study found that nurses were spending more time scurrying around and updating charts than they spent with patients.

"We found that nurses were spending their time nursing broken systems as opposed to nursing patients," says Marilyn Chow, vice president of National Patient Care Services at KP. Some nurses starting their shifts would listen to a tape recording made by an off-going nurse about the condition of certain patients. Other nurses would huddle in a conference room away from the floor—unavailable to patients—and exchange information that way.

Working in collaboration with frontline and supervisory nurses, innovation teams at KP developed a new approach to communicating patient information at shift changes, which they call the Nurse Knowledge Exchange (NKE). The heart of the process is to have oncoming and off-going nurses meet at the patient's bedside with a portable computer, enabling them to access the patient's electronic health record. Including the patient in their handoff discussion, the nurses review the care provided during the previous shift as well as the expected care needs for the upcoming shift. Patients' voices proved to be an invaluable component in this simple yet much more consistent and effective process. To pave the way for an NKE handoff process that is as crisp as possible, a sweep by nurses happens one hour before a shift change to cover a variety of other issues with patients. During this sweep nurses check in with all patients on the unit to make sure that patient needs are attended and that interruptions to the handoff process are minimized. This approach proved effective in making for a smoother handoff using the NKE process.

Another part of the NKE approach was to place a *care board* in the patient room—a simple whiteboard—listing patient care goals and upcoming procedures. This simple tool helps patients understand their care plan and what to expect regarding their daily care. It is an ever-present reminder to caregivers, patients, and their families of the specific care plan for each patient. Finally, the innovation team, working with nurses, created a database—dubbed MY BRAIN—that can produce a written report to aid in transferring information between nurses.

## NKE Spread

NKE was so obviously a better process than the existing "non-system" for shift change handoffs that it spread virally from the pilot units to other hospitals throughout KP. In a couple of hospitals, says McCarthy, float nurses who were working in an NKE pilot unit were then "going to other units and saying, 'You need to go check out what is happening in that unit. I really like the way they do shift change.' Then we had some of those float nurses go to other hospitals in that service area, and so we started getting demand virally and that is an exciting way to start off your spread."

Chow and her colleagues wanted to spread NKE as rapidly as possible. To that end, rather than implementing the new approach in one hospital at a time, KP adopted a strategy developed by senior leaders at IHI, including Bob Lloyd and Rashad Massoud, MD. This accelerated approach is explained in detail in an IHI Innovation Series white paper that also describes the background of this *framework for spread* (Massoud, Nielsen, Nolan, Schall, and Sevin, 2006). "The concept was a wave technique versus a linear technique," says Chase. "The idea was to spread initially to a few sites simultaneously, then have those [sites] serve as mentors for the next sites." Figure 7.5 depicts the idea of exponential spread and growth, where the first unit trains three additional units and, in turn, each of those three units trains another three units.

## NKE*plus*

NKE worked well in some hospitals, and very well in others. After the process had been embedded throughout much of the KP system, some innovation leaders went back and put it under a microscope. They found that in some locations the process

**Figure 7.5. Theory of Rapid Scale Up**

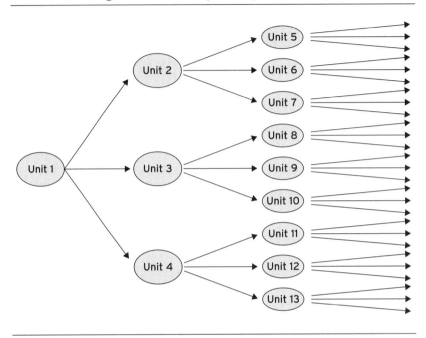

was not realizing its full potential. In particular, two problems stood out. One was the chaos that would sometimes ensue at shift change when a nurse might have to hand off her patients to as many as four other nurses. The second was that during the handoff, when nurses were together in patient rooms, there was no one available to respond to call lights, phone calls, questions from doctors, and so forth.

The innovation team engaged in idea sessions with a wide array of personnel, including frontline nurses, charge nurses, hospitalists, pharmacists, patient care technicians, unit managers, and others. They clearly saw the need to refine the NKE model by making two additions, that—together with the original NKE model—would constitute NKE*plus* (Figure 7.6).

The first new element targeted *preshift assignments*. This involved a charge nurse "assigning patients to oncoming RNs, striving for one-to-one handoffs between nurses when possible

**Figure 7.6. NKE*plus***

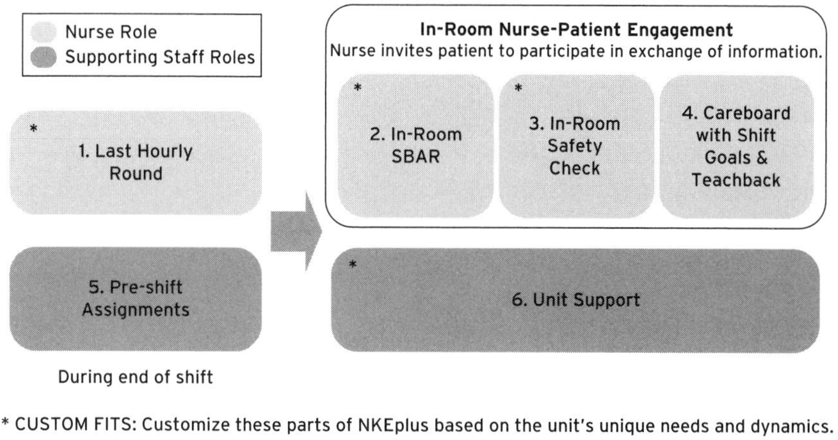

| | In-Room Nurse-Patient Engagement |
| Nurse Role | Nurse invites patient to participate in exchange of information. |
| Supporting Staff Roles | |

* 1. Last Hourly Round

* 2. In-Room SBAR

* 3. In-Room Safety Check

4. Careboard with Shift Goals & Teachback

5. Pre-shift Assignments

* 6. Unit Support

During end of shift

\* CUSTOM FITS: Customize these parts of NKEplus based on the unit's unique needs and dynamics.

*Note:* SBAR (situation-background-assessment-recommendation) is defined by IHI as a "framework for communication between members of the health care team about a patient's condition."

([one] off-going RN hands over all patients to one oncoming RN.) The off-going charge RN should work with unit clerks to get assignments clearly posted prior to shift change." This meant that "RNs are prepared to start as soon as they arrive," and they know which of the off-going nurses they will take a report from. Off-going nurses would also know to which oncoming nurses they would give their report. "By minimizing multiple handoffs between different nurses, RNs aren't 'waiting around' as much and can spend more time with patients in the room during shift changes."

The second new element involved *unit support*, which "consists of coordinating support staff and unit management to minimize disruptions to nurses during shift change." Unit support involves various activities, including using support staff and unit managers to respond to patient call lights during shift change in an effort not to distract nurses from their critically important transition work during shift handoffs.

NKE*plus* has six essential components (as shown in Figure 7.6) and is designed to produce better preparation on the unit and improved coordination among personnel.

"What is really interesting about having design infrastructure that can exist over the long term is that, five years later, we went back and picked up the pieces. . . where we left off," says McCarthy. "We implemented Nurse Knowledge Exchange across our system; it worked in many places and some places it didn't work, and so we went back and. . . did more exploration, found some details that we missed the first round, and so we redesigned it."

One result of NKE and NKE*plus* in the Sacramento and Santa Clara pilot tests was a significant increase in the amount of time nurses were able to spend at the patient bedside—a 19.6 percent increase. This translates to nearly an additional hour in a ten-hour shift.

## Developing the Garfield Health Care Innovation Center

Marilyn Chow was becoming concerned about all the work that nurses were asked to do and all the devices they were required to carry. She read about the Cleveland Clinic's Nursing Unit of the Future project and was impressed with the clinic's ability to simulate various nursing tools and processes. Chow considered what a comparable center at KP might look like. She hired Jennifer Liebermann, who had significant experience in business and in starting internal ventures, to help KP develop this idea further.

Chow and Liebermann, who would become director of the new Kaiser Permanente Sidney R. Garfield Health Care Innovation Center, began to put some thoughts together. The more they collaborated within KP, the more the scope of the project grew—from a simulation area for nurses to a simulation area for almost anything clinical-related and for architectural design, IT implementation, and home-based self-care. "We were focused on how space, technology, and workflow come together," says Liebermann. She worked with senior leaders in nursing, technology, and facilities to envision and design a new space in which to test new technology to determine whether it would actually work in hospitals and physician offices.

While planning the new Innovation Center, Jennifer Liebermann, Christi Zuber, Chris McCarthy, and Marilyn Chow visited the McDonald's simulation center, known as the Core Lab, in Chicago. The lab includes a large open space and areas where the fast-food company can create test kitchens to test the flow of workers and interactions with customers, and to examine space, technology, and workflow. "One thing I learned is how much [McDonald's pays] attention to the details," says McCarthy.

"They can pump in live data from any restaurant in the world and see how their innovations are going to react to it. They have this set-up of their space and they can figure out how many cars are coming through the drive-thru in Singapore and they can simulate that at their [lab]."

The KP team incorporated ideas from their collaborations with KP staff and from the McDonald's lab into the Garfield Health Care Innovation Center. Although many, if not most, of KP's tools and techniques for improvement and spread can be adopted by health care organizations of any size, the scope and capability of the Garfield Center is uniquely KP—and perhaps unique in all of health care. (There are other health care simulation centers, of course, including the Center for Learning and Innovation at the North Shore-Long Island Jewish Health System. With 450,000 square feet and nineteen simulation rooms, it is among the largest of such centers anywhere, and has a strong focus on teaching.)

The Garfield Center is a 37,000-square-foot structure where a wide variety of technological and workflow changes undergo simulation under real-world conditions. The Center includes a hospital ward, surgical suite, labor and delivery area, pediatric room, patient home, standard and special needs medical-surgical rooms, critical care patient room, consulting room, family waiting area, emergency department treatment room, operating room, and staff unit core areas with nurse workstations.

The purpose of the Garfield Center is, first, to simulate any new technology, design, or process that KP is considering, before applying it in any KP clinics or hospitals. The Center's prototyping zones allow teams to test ideas and evolve them rapidly, using flexible materials that can be quickly moved. The extensive hospital and clinic zones integrate space, technology, and workflow.

The home zone provides a window into Kaiser Permanente's future, where health and wellness are delivered to its members outside traditional health care facilities.

Physical activities such as enactments or role-playing allow people to see and experience new ideas, often in three dimensions. Rapid-cycle testing allows designers to "fail early and often" to get to solutions that work. In this process, designers create a learning environment where all ideas are valued and innovation can thrive.

Dr. Yan Chow, director of innovation and advanced technology at KP, says the Garfield Center allows teams to "test in as real a setting as possible without disrupting operations." He also notes that KP is now building all its hospitals to a single template—which is far more economical than a one-off approach—and that the core of that template is replicated at the Garfield Center, which means that the template can evolve in relation to the new processes and approaches that are successfully tested.

One example of these testing processes occurred during work on KP MedRite. Clinical teams were coming up with various ideas to reduce interruptions for nurses, and some pharmacists suggested the possibility of using the wireless carts—computers on wheels—that KP nurses use when making rounds of hospital wards. Pharmacists were excited about using the wireless carts because they contained a special section to hold patient medications. The theory was that nurses could carry medications with them during the course of their work and provide medications to patients without having to go back to a central medication dispensary every time. It seemed logical that the new carts could make this work more efficient, but buying thousands of carts for the entire KP system would be a large financial investment. Thus KP purchased two carts, created a simulated situation in the Garfield Center hospital ward, and brought in a team of frontline nurses to test how the carts functioned. As improvement teams and technicians gathered to observe the simulation, the nurses went about their work on the simulated hospital ward just as they would do in their normal routine.

Yan Chow says that within fifteen minutes the nurses were complaining about the new carts. Although the devices were theoretically what the nurses had asked for, in practice they did not work. First, there were ergonomic issues because, with the new heavy metal boxes for medications, the carts now weighed in excess of one hundred pounds. Second, the nurses worried about what could happen to the medication—including strictly controlled narcotic substances—if they stepped away from the carts to perform various tasks for patients. The locks on the medication boxes were too complicated to work, and the nurses felt these boxes tethered them to the carts, preventing them from stepping away.

"It was very clear to the nurses that [the carts] would not work," says Yan Chow. He says they later spoke with an official from another large health system that had purchased three thousand carts without testing them in advance—at least not in the type of real-life setting provided by the Garfield Center. The KP team later learned that the other health system had stopped using the carts.

Yan Chow believes that one of the greatest values of the Garfield Center lies in what it *prevents* KP from doing, as was the case with the carts. "It has a great value in stopping things," he says. "In innovation, sometimes failure is even more important than success."

## Looking to the Future

Dr. Jack Cochran, executive director of the Permanente Federation, the national umbrella organization representing the regional Permanente Medical Groups that together employ approximately 16,000 physicians, sees KP's progression as part of a large, historical shift in health care from "the industrial age of medicine to the information age of medicine." He says that the industrial age model in medicine—in which everything is "physician centric" and focused on the clinic visit—remains very much the status quo in much of the United States. In contrast, Cochran says, "every other industry has moved from the archaic model to the modern one." At KP, the focus for some years has been to "put the customer in the center and move into the information age."

Cochran poses two questions to help determine whether a provider is working under the industrial age model or the information age model. The first question, which has been asked for generations in medicine, is posed to a doctor: How many patients can you see today? The second question is asked of a health care team: How many patients' problems can you solve today? He talks of information age care teams made up of physicians, nurses, medical assistants, pharmacists, and others who are working together to go far beyond the traditional visit to help patients—via e-mail, e-visits, classes, and more. With electronic medical records, for example, Kaiser Permanente can sort and analyze data into registries and other data-based tools to "create a much more intense learning community so we have faster spread and get better everywhere."

Cochran notes that central to health care improvement in the information age is the determination by doctors to find new and effective ways to improve the quality of their patients' health. He points to KP's proactive office encounter program, which relies on real-time data in KP HealthConnect to find gaps in care and then quickly fill those gaps.

"When you have good data that is readily accessible you can create lists, registries, and other data sets that can then be monitored and overseen by health care teams to ensure that adequate prevention and monitoring is in place," he says. "This data enables you to see instantly [which patients are or are not] current in areas such as standard treatments for diabetes, or the need for screenings such as mammograms. If someone is overdue for a mammogram, for example, the tradition has been to send them [reminder] cards, letters, or to call them. But in [the proactive office encounter] model, we combine the learnings of supply and demand and use of mammography resources to create schedules that can be receptive to same-day arrivals of patients who are in the clinic for other reasons.

"So, with our proactive office encounter, when Mrs. Jones comes in for an eye exam, a prompt comes up to the receptionist saying Mrs. Jones needs a mammogram, and we then remind Mrs. Jones that she needs the test and we offer to do it while she is there in the office." Linking this prompt to a mammogram schedule with open appointments creates an immediate solution. The Southern California region developed the new approach because they were not satisfied with their mammography screening rates. With the new approach, they became number one in the entire country in 2008 on National Committee for Quality Assurance (NCQA) measures of patient compliance with mammograms.

Cochran says the power of the Kaiser Permanente culture to teach and learn from one another and to spread innovation is clearly indicated by the fact that the year after Southern California's success, the KP Hawaii region was number one on the NCQA mammogram ranking. And the following year the KP Georgia region was first.

Yan Chow sees a series of three macro trends as having profound impacts on health care and, in particular, on the ways in which the role of technology in health care will grow. The first trend is that the "aging population across the world is acquiring a lot more chronic conditions and that's very expensive. That trend is a huge driver of all kinds of things in technology."

The second macro trend is a looming shortage of primary care physicians. Yan Chow cites an estimate that by 2020, the United States could be short 40,000 family care physicians. Thus, he says, it is necessary for primary care to be delivered by teams, and the teams will need to have constant interaction with their patients.

This interaction will be enabled by the third macro trend— the central role of mobile phones in people's daily lives. Yan Chow envisions telehealth applications such as video visits, remote monitoring, patients transmitting information to providers, and other ways to deliver care beyond the walls of a clinic, and he believes mobile phones will bring patients and care teams closer together. He says, "[We'll be sending the message:] 'We're your health care partner,' as opposed to, 'We are only here when you get sick.'"

In early 2012, KP CEO George Halvorson sent an email to numerous KP colleagues "Celebrating Our Medical Records in the Palms of Our Hands." He wrote that

> nearly 9 million people can now get access to their medical information through their iPhones, Android devices, Blackberrys, or e-empowered mobile devices. KP.org, in other words, can now be accessed on your own phone.

That is a huge breakthrough. People with those devices can now get their lab results, refill their prescriptions, and even email their doctors using their Androids or iPhones. . .

We clearly lead the world on connectivity.

No one else can come close to having that level of convenient connectivity for their patients and members.

I have been testing the new app personally for a couple of weeks on my own iPhone. I love it. I had some blood tests run a couple weeks ago. The results were on my iPhone a couple of hours after the tests were drawn—along with our always lovely and very clear, medically literate explanation of what each test means.

After getting the tests, I exchanged a couple of emails with my doctor—asking questions and getting answers in a way that was incredibly convenient and informative. I didn't have to drive to our medical site to get that information. I had it on my phone.

Connectivity is a wonderful thing. These devices and apps are changing the world around us in many ways. Health care had not been part of the evolution. Now it is. . . .

From KP's perspective, this may well be the heart of the matter. Yan Chow is enunciating the essential KP creed—that KP is there to keep patients healthy, not just to care for them when they are ill. This is not new to KP. Although many organizations have adopted a more holistic view of health in recent years, KP launched its Total Health approach which focuses on all the lifestyle issues that have a profound impact on wellness. The intent is to keep members healthy versus caring for them only when they are sick.

"We are able to provide our members with high quality and cutting edge care, including those with challenging chronic conditions," says Bernard Tyson, president and chief operating officer of Kaiser Permanente. "With the help of technology, our medical records, and our integrated system, we are able to identify members based on criteria including ethnicity and chronic condition to focus relentlessly on prevention as well as managing the cost of care. Our work builds on our mission of providing high quality and affordable care by getting into our communities to identify opportunities where we can play a more assertive role in prevention, such as sponsoring farmer's markets in neighborhoods with limited access to fresh produce. This allows us to help foster a healthier lifestyle that leads to total health."

"When we say we want our employees, members, and communities to thrive, we really mean it," continues Tyson. "To thrive is to achieve total health—in mind, body, and spirit. At Kaiser Permanente, our mission is to help you do just that."

KP's overall performance, as measured in a variety of ways, establishes it as one of the highest performing health care organizations in the country.

- NCQA rankings indicated that the top four Medicare plans in the U.S. are within the KP universe and that KP "is ranked #1 in Medicare in each of the KP regional markets" where KP operates.
- KP ranks first in the nation in nine Medicare HEDIS measures, including breast cancer screening, weight assessment for adults, and controlling high blood pressure
- KP ranks first in the nation in 11 commercial HEDIS measures, including weight assessment for children, appropriate use of medication in asthma patients, and chlamydia screening for women.
- And KP has received the highest CMS ratings (five stars) in its California, Colorado, Hawaii, and Northwest regions.

## Keys to Doing This Work

*Christi Zuber (KP Innovation Consultancy): Keys to a Successful Improvement Journey*

- **Patience**. Be patient enough to take it one step at a time. Don't think you'll get it right the first time. Be open to learning and failure.
- **Pacing**. Don't start improvement work by tackling big, politically sensitive problems. That almost guarantees failure. You've got to learn your way to what will work for you.

*Chris McCarthy (KP Innovation Consultancy): Keys to a*
*Successful Improvement Journey*

- **Simplicity**. It is wise to keep it simple. Do some basics. You do
  not have to do a full ethnographic study, but just asking some
  very simple questions such as "What are our problems here?"
  can identify a true need or a true problem in a system.
- **An informed front line**. Sometimes the front line might not
  be exposed to a particular problem. By doing some basic
  ethnography, they and their managers can see what the
  problem is, and can say, "This is one way we can solve this
  problem."
- **Minimum specifications**. Use the concept of minimum specifications to focus the improvement work and still enable local
  adaptation.
- **Good data**. Measure. Share the data. Talk about them.
- **Branding**. Name (brand) the things that work. At KP, for
  example, nurses don't just do medication administration, they
  do KP MedRite, and because it is branded, people pay attention to it, measure it, and do leadership walk-arounds. Because
  people are people, things will drift, and then you have to
  figure out how to drift back, and it is only through measurement, walk-arounds, and paying attention that you can even
  catch the drift.
- **Recognize it's an ongoing journey**. Innovation or improvement journeys never end. They require behavioral change,
  and behavioral change is not an on-off switch; it requires
  ongoing attention.

*Jennifer Liebermann (Garfield Health Care Innovation*
*Center): Keys to Inspiring and Enabling Innovation*
*in a Large Organization*

- **Risk-taking**. Establish a climate in which people feel okay trying out new ideas. Do not shut down ideas before they've been
  vetted; demonstrate more interest in learning from failure
  than in punishing people for it.
- **Resources**. Resources need not always be concrete. Time, permission, and autonomy to innovate may be what are needed.

- **Knowledge**. Establish free-flowing information inside and outside the organization on what innovations are effective and what other organizations are working on. This will help you to see new connections between concepts.
- **Goals**. Clearly defined aspirational goals signal that innovation is important.
- **Rewards**. Offer rewards for innovation. Two proven incentives are more autonomy to innovate and professional development opportunities that support an innovator's career path.
- **Recognition**. Offer recognition for innovation. For example, giving individuals a chance to share their innovations with a larger group (as KP does through the Garfield Innovation Network) is a powerful form of recognition.
- **Tools**. Give people a set of tools with which they can innovate. Examples include the simulation areas at the Garfield Health Care Innovation Center; the IDEO-inspired, human-centered design methodology; and the IHI metrics methodology used by KP's Innovation Consultancy.
- **Relationships**. An innovative culture fosters relationships among people. Research shows that innovation is rarely the product of a lone genius—instead it arises when people's diverse and divergent opinions come together in a holistic solution to a problem [adapted from Liebermann, 2010].

# 8

# No Excuses

## Effective Leadership to Achieve the Triple Aim

Jim Conway, former chief operating officer at the Dana Farber Cancer Institute and IHI Senior Fellow, is often quoted asking, *"If you knew, why didn't you do?"* This challenge to change reaches to the heart of professionalism for providers and leaders. And though there are examples of the rapid spread of new health care technology or surgical methods, health care has been notoriously slow in doing precisely what Jim Conway suggests: to insist on the rapid, nimble adoption of techniques and practices that demonstrably result in better care for individuals and populations and lower costs and to provide the leadership support to make that possible. The subtext of Jim's comment is simple: There are no excuses for leaders failing to pursue this path.

The pursuit of the Triple Aim requires a new kind of leadership. In health care, this is a turbulent time of many challenges and frustrations. But it is also a remarkable period of excitement, innovation, and opportunity to transform our system into one that performs far more effectively on quality and cost. This is a time when health care leaders need new skills and competencies in order to serve as effective stewards of change and reform.

The innovations developed to pursue the Triple Aim that are described in this book demonstrate that reform is not only possible but flourishing in a wide variety of organizations throughout the country. *In each case, the key driver of successful innovation and change is effective, often visionary, leadership.* The leaders we write about—and many others, as well—are not waiting to see what the new health care landscape will look like beyond the horizon. They are acting in bold ways both to improve their organizations today and to position them effectively for the years ahead.

Without waiting for a national change in payment systems, for example, these organizations are implementing forward-thinking models. Some of these models might present a financial challenge in the short term but they allow providers to keep the promise to patients that their care will be integrated, coordinated, evidence based, and centered in their preferences and needs. These new models also hold the promise that health of the system and the community will be improved by better monitoring of data, the development of proactive clinical encounters of all kinds (office visits, e-mails, telephone consultations, group education sessions), and the control of per capita costs. To spread these local successes nationally, we need more of the kind of leadership demonstrated in these stories.

## The Leader's Role in Spread

Tom Nolan spells out the leader's role in improvement as building will, generating or finding better ideas and models, and engaging in impeccable execution. How have the leaders in the innovative systems we have discussed demonstrated will, ideas, and execution, and how can people in health care from the executive offices to the front lines learn how to accelerate the transfer of best practices to all?

### Will

Building will starts with boards of directors and leaders understanding the results of today's performance. The static red, yellow, and green dashboards reviewed at many leadership meetings are reliable only in their failure to build will. Too often, they fail to convey the reality of care in an institution, thus falsely assuring leaders that their organization's quality results are exemplary.

We propose four questions that every leadership team should answer and, through that exercise, build the will required to undertake the challenging work of innovation and cultural change:

- Do you know how good your organization is?
- Do you know where your organization stands relative to the best?
- Do you know where variation exists in your organization?
- Do you know your organization's rate of improvement over time?

### Do You Know How Good Your Organization Is?

Leaders like Mary Brainerd at HealthPartners use several methods for answering the question about organizational performance. They look at data at the level of the individual (for example, a diabetes measure that can be compared to an optimal measure) and at the level of the population (for example, for all the patients with diabetes in a practice), and then compare those findings with national guidelines (for example, those from the Institute for Clinical Systems Improvement). A balanced portfolio of metrics is key to the leader's ability to answer this question, and Triple Aim metrics can provide a wide view of quality, health, and cost.

As important as the numbers are, the stories behind them are even more vital to a leader's understanding of performance. Dr. Tony DiGioia's use of students and caregivers to shadow the patient journey produced valuable intelligence on process failures, handover problems, waste, and complications that would never show up on a balanced scorecard. Dr. Bob Mecklenburg's meetings with Annette King to discuss health care value for Starbucks employees brought to light process failures, higher-than-market costs, and the burden of absenteeism from low back pain. At CareOregon, seeing a room filled with homeless men and women suffering from addictions, now listening to peaceful music and being treated with acupuncture, offers insight into pursuing the Triple Aim with a challenging population.

The stories show that building will means getting out to the front lines—going to the *gemba* in lean management terminology. It is

urgent that leaders facing financial challenges requiring budget cuts
see the impact of these changes at the point of care. This book is
filled with examples of better care at a lower cost, but when budget
cuts happen in isolation from care redesign, looking only at score-
cards can dupe leaders into believing that quality is unaffected. And
building will is key at all levels in an organization. Many board meetings at health care organizations now start with a story of a patient
exceptionally cared for or one who suffered harm through system
failures. Most board members can now interpret clinical data, and
boards spend as much time on the quality of care as they historically
spent on financial stability, acquisitions, and construction projects.

Senior teams are building will by rounding in care settings,
talking with staff and patients, and reviewing reports together.
The understanding that results leads to change. For example,
chief financial officers like Scott Hamlin at Cincinnati Children's
Hospital Medical Center know that costs can be reduced when
flow through the hospital is optimized, and Hamlin's work with
Dr. Uma Kotagal has enabled the hospital to optimize getting
every patient in the right place with the right staff at the right
time. And Kotagal understands the financial savings associated
with the reduction of health care–associated infections.

Frontline managers build will best when they connect care
providers and workers with the meaning of the work to patients
and families. When a hospital CEO invited the staff from central
sterile processing to observe a procedure in the operating room,
one of these staffers was moved to tears by seeing how her work
was applied and how it mattered in the OR setting. The experience moved her from thinking of herself as a technical processor
to thinking of herself as a part of the care team.

Outside the pathology lab at Gundersen Lutheran Hospital
in La Crosse, Wisconsin, there is a photo of a vibrant young man
named John. Next to his picture on one side, his words tell the
story of his cancer and treatment and, on the other side, photos
of the cells that were present on his pathology slides reveal his
diagnosis. Pathologist Dan Schreith invited John to visit the lab,
and the staff described the meaning they found in their work
from meeting the patient behind the slides.

Building will is often overlooked or considered unnecessary
in health care settings—where caregivers come to such important

work each day—but many frontline staff today are feeling overwhelmed, rushed, and disempowered. Innovation and improvement in these settings needs to start with seeing the gaps that exist and then building the capabilities to change performance for the better.

### Do You Know Where Your Organization Stands Relative to the Best?

The most innovative leaders keep their eyes on true north by looking to the best for comparative results and new ideas. With Hospital Compare from Medicare, statewide comparative databases like Minnesota Community Measurement, and the ability to gather and analyze many layers of financial and health data as Blue Cross Blue Shield of Massachusetts does in administering the Alternative Quality Contract, leaders and clinicians can see how their results compare to the best in multiple areas, and each gap revealed is a true will-building mechanism. The days of excusing gaps by claiming that "my patients are sicker" are past, as clinicians and leaders seek answers to the comparative question. When boards raise the issue of their organization's relative performance, the will to learn and change accelerates at all levels.

One way that leaders show the gap between current performance and the best is the *live case visit* method for learning. David Garvin of the Harvard Business School describes this method as a powerful tool for learning about comparative quality (Maureen Bisognano, 2011, pers. comm.), and we have found it a highly engaging and effective way for frontline teams to move quality and cost metrics efficiently. In the live case visit method, leaders identify an area for improvement and find an organization with superior or best performance in that balanced set of dimensions. Prior to the visit, the staff who will visit this organization study their own internal processes by, for example, evaluating the overall cost, quality outcomes, service dimensions, and staff vitality for the care for patients requiring continuous care for chronic disease or for a surgical service.

The visitors then make a site visit to the better performing organization (the host), and staff at the host describe how they have managed and improved care for this patient group. (The process is much like the approach CareOregon used when traveling to learn at Southcentral Foundation in Anchorage, described in Chapter Three.) The visitors break into small groups and walk the *gemba*. They interview host staff and learn how they have managed the innovations and improvements in care. The visitors reflect on the challenges they experience back at home, and the host staff describe how they have worked with similar challenges, such as persuading resistant professionals, optimizing supply management, or connecting various providers to accomplish seamless care for patients. After the visitors take some time to regroup and design the strategy they will apply on their return home, they meet again with the host staff and share their plans. The day ends with the visitors reflecting back to the host staff their perceptions of how the host organization really improves. They share what they have understood about the supports and the challenges and the ways in which the host organization has overcome the barriers to driving substantial change. We have seen improvements in sites quickly after a visitor team returns home, and interestingly the host organization benefits as well. Through the live case visit process, the senior leaders of the host organization develop a better understanding of where they have ready capability and experience with improvement.

### Do You Know Where Variation Exists in Your Organization?

When the leaders at Virginia Mason Medical Center and at HealthPartners drilled down into their data, they found variation within their organization's practice patterns, much of it resulting from historical habits and routines in care processes. Such variation is ubiquitous and often hides opportunities for learning from the best practices within the system. When leaders have detailed information on quality process and outcome measures as well as costs, they can stimulate learning dialogues and use the data not for judgment but for improvement. When leaders cannot see the variation, or when they develop a tolerance for "to each his own" care practices, patients receive varying levels of care and costs are excessive.

In a recent conversation with Captain Chesley "Sully" Sullenberger (personal communication)—known for his safe emergency landing of US Airways Flight 1549 on the Hudson River after a crippling encounter with a flock of geese—he relayed the history of safety improvements in aviation and pointed to a change in aviation culture that had the specific goal of reducing variation as a key lever for improving safety. Sullenberger described his early days as a pilot, and talked about the "pilot preference list" that each copilot carried to ensure a readiness to comport with the idiosyncrasies of each pilot. Each flight was adjusted to the specific processes of the pilot, much as many operating room staff carry *physician preference cards* and constantly change processes to accord with the individual habits of each surgeon. The variation in these situations is not defined by the unique needs of the patient, but by the varying methods of the staff.

Sullenberger noted that safety requires standardization of routine processes so that pilots can be prepared to react to unforeseen circumstances (such as birds flying into and shutting down airplane engines), and he described how airline leaders, pilots' union leaders, and copilots all combined forces to change the culture to one reliant on standardization as a means to improve safety. Only when a few respected pilots changed their own ways of practice and began to share their sense of better safety, did the whole industry mobilize to change. Recognizing variation in health care organizations is similarly a step toward building the will to change the culture so it supports standardization and thus reliability.

### Do You Know Your Organization's Rate of Improvement over Time?
Leaders and boards often look at quarterly or annual metrics on cost and quality, and they assume that they are improving year on year. A helpful exercise for the senior team is to ask each member to estimate the trends in the key metrics over the last five years, and then to compare the estimates to the actual rates of improvement over time. In many cases, seeing stagnant results and small improvements prompts deep conversations about aims and energizes support for building improvement capability and more.

When leaders want to ensure reliable change in performance, they look to identify the system that could produce the desired outcome. After the leaders at Palmetto Health in Columbia, South Carolina, moved from looking at static mortality rates to examining hospital standardized mortality ratios

(HSMRs) over time, they focused on building a driver diagram that defined the systems they would need to work on to reduce mortality across their hospitals. Such a diagram serves as a picture of the system and links the desired outcome with key drivers—primary and secondary levers (see Figure 8.1 for an example). Leaders find these system maps helpful in many ways but particularly because they break down the complexities of organizing improvement for an outcome measure, spelling out what needs attention.

The leaders at Palmetto Health organized improvement teams in several areas simultaneously (the OR, intensive care units, ED, and medical-surgical units). This portfolio of projects, chartered and led by the system's leaders, produced dramatic and sustained change as the leaders took on the system as a whole, piloted and implemented changes, and then spread the new models throughout Palmetto.

### Figure 8.1. Mortality Reduction Driver Diagram

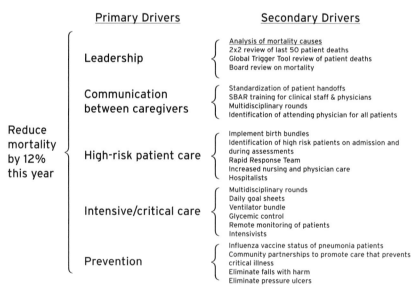

*Note:* SBAR in this figure refers to "Situation, Background, Assessment, Recommendation"—a communication tool.

## Ideas

When CareOregon's medical director Dr. David Labby and CEO Dave Ford visited Southcentral Foundation in Anchorage, Alaska, they learned to see in a new way. Familiar work done in completely new ways inspired them to develop change concepts they would test with providers back in Portland. Bellin Health CEO George Kerwin was enthusiastic about making progress on the Triple Aim for employees, and started with improving care for his own organization's staff. Whether the new ways to see come from a visit to another state, from shadowing a patient's journey across a complex system, or from your own staff, new models of care are essential for achieving better results at a lower cost.

Ideas can come from seeing the journey of a patient across sites or from interviewing patients to understand both the burden of an illness and the burden of a treatment. One helpful exercise, based on the work of Dr. David Gustafson at the University of Wisconsin-Madison, engages leaders and providers at all levels in interviewing a patient or family member in a structured way. A family physician, for example, interviewed the mother of a child with asthma, and began the interview by asking, "What is it like to have a young son with asthma?" The mother recounted struggles with her husband who continued to smoke at home, stress over missing work due to exacerbations in her son's condition, and fear of being fired. She talked about her concerns for her son's sense of foreboding, with the asthma flare-ups causing him a great deal of stress and fear in addition to the physical symptoms. The financial burden of medication and co-pays, on top of her fear that she would lose insurance coverage if she lost her job, was a central part of the conversation. The mother said, "Every day, I am on pins and needles." The physician then asked about her encounters with the health system and the conversation took an unexpected turn. The mother noted challenges in getting appointments that didn't force her to miss work. She said she worried that she did not always understanding the complex language of care. She described the usual visit and phone call with the staff and the interviewer noted that her concerns were never raised in these encounters. The interviewer asked if the mother's team knew about her concerns, and

## SAMPLE INTERVIEW FORM

1. Identify a patient (or family caregiver) who is bright and insightful and who has experienced a long-term or serious health care concern. For your first effort at an interview, you might select a relative or friend of yours: for example, an aunt who was the caregiver of a person with Alzheimer's or a friend who is a cancer survivor.

2. Schedule a forty-five-minute time to interview the person, either in person or by telephone.

3. Begin by asking the person to think broadly about his or her situation. Then ask the person to talk about what it is like to be in that situation with his or her particular disease or health concern. How does it affect the person's life? What are the main fears, frustrations, inconveniences, and uncertainties he or she faces? What makes it hard to be in this situation? What helps the person overcome difficulties in dealing with the situation?

4. Now, move to health care–specific issues. Ask the person to think about a specific time when health was a problem and when he or she saw a health care provider about it. Ask the person to describe the time in specific detail. What were the fears, frustrations, inconveniences, and uncertainties? What did he or she wish had happened that did not happen? What was the hardest part about being a patient in the health care system? What positive surprises did he or she experience?

   • Do let the person talk and move off into other health and life events if he or she wishes. Be mindful of and try to minimize interruptions. Follow up for details when the responses are general. When the person finishes describing one health event, move on to another, until he or she runs out of steam.

   • Do not defend yourself or the health care system. You are there to learn. You are not there to explain, teach, or be judgmental.

5. When you have completed the interview, compile the results into a list of needs, noting each need only once. Then group these needs into categories on the basis of key similarities and label each category. Finish by writing up your thoughts about how the interview went and what could have made it go better. What made it challenging or worthwhile? What did you learn that you could carry over to quality improvement work? Your narrative should be no longer than one to two pages.

she said that these issues had not been discussed and that the visits focused on the child's test results and clinical needs.

Having physicians and staff conduct an interview like this is a powerful tool to prompt new ideas for care systems, as in the sample interview form supplied here.

The leaders with the best track records for innovation have established systems and structures for building innovative ideas or searching them out. Dr. William Rupp, the CEO of the Mayo Clinic in Jacksonville, Florida, has his own specific methods for bringing ideas into the system. He purchased subscriptions for all key journals for clinicians who brought the latest and best research to the right teams in the hospital in a timely way. He allocated time for a clinical pharmacist to scan relevant Web sites and journals each week, and would then bring the new information to the appropriate committees and leaders. This structured process for scanning and responding apace also led Rupp to support the attendance of dozens of clinicians at key conferences each year, with the specific assignment to scan for and return with new ideas to improve care.

John O'Brien, the CEO of UMass Memorial Health Care, has used a monthly breakfast to get new ideas. He has invited all employees who have been patients or have had family members as patients in the system that month to a breakfast and asked them this key question: "What rules did you have to break to make your care better?" Knowing that his staff members have access to knowledge and systems and can therefore break the rules, the list that is generated served as O'Brien's agenda for implementing new ideas that improve care for all.

Another way to prompt improvement teams to develop new ideas is a method that design firm IDEO calls a *deep dive*, where teams go into the field and use anthropological tools to look at care across a journey. New improvement teams might begin their design journey by consulting this list of general change concepts from *The Improvement Guide, Second Edition,* by Langley, Moen, Nolan, Nolan, Norman, and Provost (2009 p. 359):

1. Eliminate things that are not used
2. Eliminate multiple entry
3. Reduce or eliminate overkill
4. Reduce controls on the system
5. Recycle or reuse
6. Use substitution
7. Reduce classification
8. Remove intermediaries
9. Match the amount to the need
10. Use sampling
11. Change targets or set points
12. Synchronize
13. Schedule into multiple processes
14. Minimize handoffs
15. Move steps in the process close together
16. Find and remove bottlenecks
17. Use automation
18. Smooth workflow
19. Do tasks in parallel
20. Consider people as in the same system
21. Use multiple processing units
22. Adjust to peak demand
23. Match inventory to predicted demand
24. Use pull systems
25. Reduce choice of features
26. Reduce multiple brands of the same item
27. Give people access to information
28. Use proper measurements
29. Take care of basics
30. Reduce demotivating aspects of the pay system

31. Conduct training
32. Implement cross-training
33. Invest more resources in improvement
34. Focus on core process and purpose
35. Share risks
36. Emphasize natural and logical consequences
37. Develop alliances and cooperative relationships
38. Listen to customers
39. Coach the customer to use a product/service
40. Focus on the outcome to a customer
41. Use a coordinator
42. Reach an agreement on expectations
43. Outsource for "free"
44. Optimize level of inspection
45. Work with suppliers
46. Reduce setup or startup time
47. Set up timing to use discounts
48. Optimize maintenance
49. Extend specialist's time
50. Reduce wait time
51. Standardization (create a formal process)
52. Stop tampering
53. Develop operational definitions
54. Improve predictions
55. Develop contingency plans
56. Sort product into grades
57. Desensitize
58. Exploit variation
59. Use reminders
60. Use differentiation
61. Use constraints
62. Use affordances
63. Mass customize
64. Offer product/service anytime
65. Offer product/service anyplace
66. Emphasize intangibles
67. Influence or take advantage of fashion trends
68. Reduce the number of components
69. Disguise defects or problems
70. Differentiate product using quality dimensions
71. Change the order of process steps
72. Manage uncertainty, not tasks

## Execution

Tom Nolan, in the 2007 IHI white paper *Execution of Strategic Improvement Initiatives to Produce System-Level Results,* describes organizations with a proven track record in system-level improvement and defines their capabilities in three key areas: (1) the ability to consistently deliver on *system-level aims,* (2) strong and ever-present *local management and supervision,* and (3) the *development* of enough employees to create a cadre of leaders devoted to improvement.

Most of the leaders discussed in this book took the bold step of setting the Triple Aim as their system-level goal. Leadership for the Triple Aim requires that leaders see the population they serve and understand their organization's performance on health, care, and cost (Figure 8.2).

These leaders sponsor a portfolio of projects intended to test new ideas and models under local control and specified circumstances. When Dr. Brian Rank and colleagues started the Care Model Process at HealthPartners, he began by testing

### Figure 8.2. Triple Aim System Design

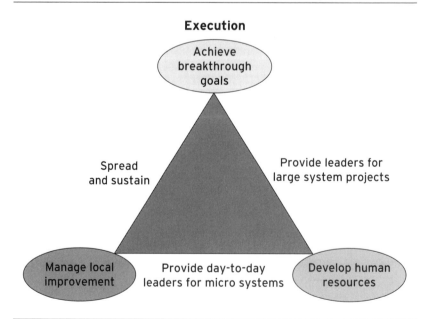

the components and the system of the model in one setting, then made it part of daily operations in that setting, and then refined it in ways that would ensure success in other settings and accelerate spread. The following description of these three stages is adapted from *The Improvement Guide, Second Edition* (Langley et al., 2009).

- **Testing.** Trying and adapting ideas on a small scale in a pilot population. Learning how to make the idea work in your system.

    Change is not permanent.
    Failures are very useful here, even expected.
    Fewer people are affected than during implementation.

- **Implementing.** Making this change a part of the routine day-to-day operation of the system for your pilot population.

    Don't expect failure here.
    Design or redesign supporting processes to maintain the
        change (feedback and measurement systems, job descrip-
        tions, procedures, new employee training, and so forth.)
    More people are affected than during testing.
    Increased resistance is encountered compared to testing.
    More time is generally required for this stage than for
        testing.

- **Spreading.** Adapting changes to areas or populations other than the pilot population.

Supporting this testing-implementation-spread model requires the continual development of improvement capabilities in staff. At IHI, we use an approach called *all-teach, all-learn*. It rests on the belief that change is only spreadable and sustainable when there are enough people, with the right skills, to steward improvement and make it routine. W. Edwards Deming is often quoted as saying that "quality is everyone's responsibility" and we believe improvement is as well. Leaders need to create time and opportunities for their staff to learn the science of improvement and make it part of their daily work—to integrate within the DNA of the organization as Kaiser Permanente has done with improvement and the capacity to spread change and innovation. A continuously improving organization is a learning organization, and the future of health care is being led by these kinds of organizations.

## The Leader's Role in Changing the Culture

Building a new culture is the key driver for success in pursuing the Triple Aim. In a column for HBR Blog Network, Nilofer Merchant (2011) observed—as the title of her article suggests—"Culture Trumps Strategy, Every Time." At IHI, this cultural emphasis has long been an article of faith. As you have read in this book, culture change is hard work. It challenges deeply held beliefs and often pushes people well out of their comfort zones. It also—nearly invariably—triggers pushback. Some of that is passive-aggressive—doctors who urge one another to "wait it out" believing that the current change is a "flavor of the month." Some of the pushback is more aggressive, as Dr. Gary Kaplan experienced in the early days applying the Toyota Production System to the management of Virginia Mason Medical Center. But when leaders persist, change happens. Early adopters sign on and soon positive results bring more and more of the uncommitted over to a different cultural perspective.

As difficult as it is, however, cultural change can be liberating, inspiring, and can help restore and enhance the joy all health care professionals can take from their work. We can think of no more important aspect of leadership than creating and maintaining an effective culture.

From their first days of medical school or nursing school, professionals are taught that their patients' lives depend on their personal skill and expertise, that "if in doubt, do more." They are also taught that care happens in visits and procedures. Although the value of skill and expertise will never diminish, health care leaders will need to create and cultivate a new culture that considers care not just in visits in procedures, but across a wide continuum. Improvements of any kind—safety, reliability, throughput, waste reduction, anything—is sustainable only if the right culture exists.

Culture change to drive new models of care needs deliberate time, attention, and modeling from the senior team. Leaders can begin the journey to a new culture by first defining the new state, and exemplifying the needed changes personally and through stories.

Unfortunately, there isn't one universal "right" culture—the job of leadership would be much easier if there were. Finding the right culture depends on the unique circumstances of your organization. But any successful organizational culture should rest on a foundation of openness, effective communication, and teamwork. When leaders of organizations engaged in IHI's 100,000 Lives Campaign began their work to improve patient safety and reduce mortality, many of them instituted safety walk-arounds—regular trips to the front lines to walk in the footsteps of clinicians (and patients) and elicit input from staff. The conversations they had with staff focused on their concerns with potential risks. Often the leaders met with reassurances that managers and staff "have everything under control," but with careful and patient prodding, followed up with supportive action, staff did begin to surface potential problems. We wrote about such a situation in Chapter Seven when we described Chris McCarthy's meetings with nurses who said that everything was fine with the process of medication administration on the hospital ward. But as Chris and his colleagues probed, they found serious holes in the process—which they subsequently succeeding in filling. Some said, "I'm concerned that we are short of supply" or "I'm meeting with resistance to adopting the new procedures." Seeking out, listening, and most important, following up on voiced concerns models a new behavior and creates and reinforces a culture that empowers staff to be agents of improvement. This kind of culture strengthens connections between frontline staff and senior leadership, which enhances teamwork and belief that change, even difficult change, is possible.

Leading any health care organization to new cultural terrain is an enormous challenge. It requires fresh behaviors and technical methods that demonstrate how to thrive in a new environment. On the behavioral side, one of the biggest challenges to culture change comes from the diversity of the workforce—from professional training and backgrounds to the age distribution of the staff. Leadership approaches that are effective with physicians may need modification if they are to work for other caregivers and administrators, even as the culture moves to one where teamwork is the norm. Successful models for working with different generations require flexible and adaptable approaches. The cultural approaches that work with the generation in their mid-fifties include a sense of duty, a vision of personal achievement through hard work, and a willingness to take on new challenges for the good of the whole. The next generation (mid-twenties) are often driven by a sense of personal development, optimizing their skills and abilities, and contributing where they clearly add value and get a sense of achievement and personal growth. Finding the right balance and creating the right pathways for effective communication among different generations and groups is essential to creating the right culture.

Creating a culture of teamwork requires a vision from the leaders, crafted in stories, and supported by data that show that teamwork produces safer, more effective, and more efficient care. If successful, a culture of teamwork supports and improves joy in work in almost any setting. With a clear and compelling vision of effective teamwork, leaders can model the new culture through their own actions, often through changes in their own schedules and work. This modeling defines the change for all staff and gives them a guide to adapting themselves.

## A Broader Community-wide View

No one organization, not even a major health system or health plan, can achieve the Triple Aim alone. It requires a new kind of community coalition that connects all of the community or regional leaders in the health systems to join with public health leaders, educational and civic, to agree on aims and to form a new way to work together on health. In Memphis, for example, at the Healthy Memphis Common Table, one of the church leaders who cares for the souls of thousands of people in Memphis recently told the doctors in the coalition, "You see the patients with diabetes for fifteen minutes, twice a year, and I see the people with diabetes every week. I'll invite them to dinner at the church every Wednesday night and we'll together teach them how to get to better health."

This broader view of how to have an impact on the health of a community is in line with the work Vinod Sahney, former

IHI board chair and current IHI senior fellow, and others are doing in West Bloomfield, Michigan. Vin Sahney was designing a new hospital for the Henry Ford Health System—a new hospital that looks like no other. The leaders there have built a test kitchen and hired a world class chef to teach the community how to select healthy foods, how to cook for better health, and more. The hospital includes places to play cards and socialize for the elders in the community and a spa with yoga classes that teach self-efficacy and calm. This requires a new and wider view of health and new coalitions that are not easy to build in these fast-paced and competitive times. The skills of coalition building, perhaps learned from Marshall Ganz, senior lecturer in Public Policy at the Harvard Kennedy School, or other leaders who inspire us to think more broadly than the walls of the organizations we lead, will help, but the challenges are there.

On the technical side, leaders need specific skills and methods to create the right culture for improvement. An example of these skills is patient-centered design—a method for channeling the voices of patients and families into care processes and physical plant design more reliably. When Göran Henriks in Jönköping, Sweden, wanted to model a move to a more patient-driven culture, he invented a hypothetical patient—"Esther"—and used her story to redesign the care system across specialties and organizations. At Göran's improvement institute, Qulturum, he convened clinicians and leaders from all parts of the health system to create "Esther," a seventy-eight-year-old woman with congestive heart failure (CHF), who lives alone and is fairly independent. Göran asked the emergency medical technicians to "tell me about Esther." Using their knowledge of CHF, they answered that "Esther calls three times a year, usually at night, because she is having trouble breathing. We respond, take her vital signs, give her oxygen, and because she lives alone, we bring her to the emergency department." Göran then asks, "what's next?" turning to the emergency physicians who pick up her care. Each team knew Esther's care from their perspective, informed by their interactions, but none knew the whole journey. They all used Esther as an opportunity to redesign care throughout a patient's journey, to dive into population-level data and redesign clinical guidelines, and to build a culture of interdependent teamwork, patient centeredness, effective handovers, and reliable information systems.

Creating a culture of teamwork and open communication also requires new techniques. One example is the huddle. Effective huddles are characterized by their frequency (often), their duration (short), and their degree of collaboration (high). An example of how leaders at Cincinnati Children's Hospital use huddles is included in the Epilogue.

IHI's work on patient safety over the years has revealed that the safest health care facilities are those that have developed a *culture of safety*. Again, there are specific techniques for fostering and maintaining this culture, and foundational to any effort is a leader's clear, demonstrable commitment. This commitment is demonstrated by providing the resources, tools, and environment that all work together to ensure safety. Some of the tools that are commonly used are a reporting system for adverse events and conditions that staff believe could lead to problems. Simulations of adverse events can help staff learn the warning signs and most effective methods to mitigate harm. Resources like dedicated patient safety officers or other patient safety "champions" contribute to a culture of safety through their specific focus and responsibilities. Involving patients in care redesign projects reinforces the human aspect of patient safety and drives home the notion that harm doesn't occur in a vacuum; it affects people.

The techniques and tools to create culture change are numerous, and all leaders need to select the ones most appropriate to them and their setting. Culture may be hard to define but it is nonetheless tangible. Places with unique, effective cultures just *feel* different. Modeling and embodying the culture you want is perhaps the most important duty of a health care leader today. To paraphrase Mohandas Gandhi, leaders must *be* the change they wish to see.

We titled this chapter "No Excuses" not because we expect leaders to have a list of reasons at the ready for why their organizations can't accomplish what the innovators in this book have done but rather because we've seen the challenges leaders face *and* we've seen so many innovative and inspiring solutions. Pursuing the Triple Aim is, we believe, the right goal for everyone in health care. We hope that we've been able to provide some practical advice for leaders who believe as we do.

# Epilogue

## Innovation Everywhere

The stories presented in this book are, among other things, meant to inspire. The variety, creativity, broad applicability, and results of the projects we've described should reaffirm confidence that this nation's health care system can be transformed. But if these examples were representative of just a few pockets of innovation and excellence, if these pioneers and champions were among just a small group of like-minded people and organizations, confidence in change would wither. Luckily for all of us, they are not. The movement to transform health care and to dramatically improve quality and value grows every year. Once on the periphery, quality improvement has pervaded every corner of the system. In the more than ten years since *To Err Is Human* and *Crossing the Quality Chasm* achieved national attention, health care has gotten safer, and it has gotten better. With runaway costs now recognized as an obstacle that cannot be ignored innovators are turning their attention to value, more and more each day. What's genuinely exciting about this movement is that organizations all over this country and all over the world are working tirelessly to improve care, improve health, and increase value. What follows is a brief assemblage of additional examples of this work. A collection like this can never be exhaustive, but we offer here sketches of a further baker's dozen of some of the more promising innovations occurring in health care today.

## Collaborative Care: ThedaCare

ThedaCare, in Appleton, Wisconsin, has long been at the forefront of innovation and improvement in health care. It has developed an internal process—the ThedaCare Improvement System—used to address longstanding issues in inpatient hospital care. Leaders and staff have been vigilant in driving out waste and improving safety. In 2006, ThedaCare was selected to participate as a pilot site in the Transforming Care at the Bedside (TCAB) initiative (funded by the Robert Wood Johnson Foundation and led by the Institute for Healthcare Improvement). In conjunction with TCAB and using the ThedaCare Improvement System, the organization developed a simple but highly effective model for patient care dubbed *collaborative care*. Under the collaborative care model, each patient is seen within ninety minutes of admission by a team of clinicians—a doctor, nurse, and pharmacist—who all meet with the patient at the same time. The patient's history is determined, his chart and records are examined, and the patient or his family (or both) talks with the care team about his condition just once; there is no need to repeat the information multiple times. The three-member care team then immediately discusses the patient's condition or conditions (often right there with the patient) and agrees on a treatment plan. The plan is segmented by what staff at ThedaCare call *tollgates*—milestones managed by the nurse. The tollgates create clear, timely expectations for both the patient and provider. Once the plan is shared and clearly explained to everyone—clinicians, patient, and family members—treatment begins.

The collaborative care model ensures a comprehensive care plan understood by the patient, his family, and his provider. This direct, open communication cuts down on the ambiguity and contradictions that can plague less cooperatively delivered care. It decreases the amount of time needed by individual clinicians to review paperwork, which increases the amount of time allotted for direct interaction with patients. And it makes care better. Patient and provider satisfaction both improve using this model. Fewer medication errors are made, and hospital stays are shortened.

The model has a physical component, too. Through testing the model, ThedaCare staff found that simple yet high-impact changes to the physical space in the hospital supported the collaborative care improvements. Central nursing stations were replaced with individual workstations nearer to patient rooms. Computers were placed next to patients' beds to facilitate electronic record keeping and use. Medications and supplies were also moved to the bedside to cut down the risk of errors, and reduce the time wasted by hunting for supplies.

The results of the pilot-testing were so encouraging that collaborative care is being spread throughout the ThedaCare system. This simple model can be used almost anywhere. And the idea of collaborative, team-based care has huge potential outside the hospital. Team-based primary care is being tested all over the country, and the benefits to communication and coordination will be felt even more strongly in that part of the care system.

To learn more about collaborative care visit the Web site of the newly formed ThedaCare Center for Healthcare Value at www.createhealthcarevalue.com.

## Structured Huddles: Cincinnati Children's Hospital Medical Center

Communication breakdowns can be deadly in health care. Careful coordination of complex medication and treatment plans is essential to providing high-quality, high-value care. As the patient population grows older and the prevalence of multiple conditions in patients increases, effective communication about care has never been more crucial. Cincinnati Children's Hospital Medical Center (CCHMC), in Cincinnati, Ohio, has been testing a simple improvement—a *structured huddle*. Huddles are effective communication vehicles because they are short, fast, frequent, and highly collaborative. Their purpose is simple—ensure that everyone is on the same page before a care interaction.

At CCHMC, structured huddles are prerounding activities that involve all the caregivers who will interact with the patient. The first huddle commences at 5:30 AM and involves all the operational managers. They try to anticipate what the day will bring by examining everything: staffing, equipment needs, logistical challenges, even the weather forecast. At 7:00 AM the nurses huddle to prepare for their day. They quickly review all pertinent information to anticipate expected demand and throughput. They look at the clinical alerts for that day and plan for discharges, potential admissions, and staffing numbers to maximize one-to-one care for all patients. They also discuss the special social and clinical needs of patients to ensure patient-centered care. At 2:15 PM the leaders of every service gather for a huddle to start planning for the next day. They examine what's happened up to that point to help predict the end of the current day and identify what is crucial for the next. The last huddle of the day actually occurs in the early morning hours of the next day. At 1:00 AM the clinicians review all patient records, with special attention to patients who are or might be unstable overnight. They review the events of the day, looking for challenges that emerged and that could be prevented in the future. By mandating regular, structured, coordinated huddles, the staff at CCHMC greatly reduce the risks posed by breakdowns in communications.

## Reducing Variation: Intermountain Healthcare

For decades now, increasing value has been central to the purpose of Intermountain Healthcare in Salt Lake City, Utah. The short version of the organization's mission statement reads, "the best clinical result at the lowest necessary cost," and one can hardly imagine a simpler description of health care value. Innovators at Intermountain long ago studied the work of the great quality pioneer W. Edwards Deming, and they have adhered to his principle that the best way to reduce costs is to improve value. Starting in the mid-1980s, leaders at Intermountain began looking at clinical variation in their hospitals. Again, they did so with Deming echoing in their ears—"variation is always the enemy" was another of Deming's principles. Clinical variation, meaning differences in care delivery for what is essentially the same medical condition, was already known to be a problem. Yet many simply ascribed it to the differences among physicians and care sites. Intermountain chose to look at process variation rather than provider variation, and what it found sent the organization on a path toward true transformation of how it delivered care. A thorough review of patient records revealed that most admissions for a specific treatment had similar characteristics. But the variation in the ways the physicians administered the treatments was significant. By smoothing out that variation, costs fell and clinical outcomes stayed steady or in some instances even improved.

For example, a physician at Intermountain's LDS Hospital reduced variation in the treatment of acute respiratory distress by integrating a standardized, evidence-based care plan into the normal workflow for all physicians, thus making this one care protocol the normative default. Results were astonishing. Variance from evidence-based guidelines dropped from 59 percent to 6 percent, patient survival increased from 9.5 percent to 44 percent, the time it took physicians to administer the treatment was halved, and the total cost of care was reduced 25 percent.

To spread similar results to other processes and conditions, Intermountain instituted a process of *clinical integration.* It began with identifying the key clinical processes that the health system delivered. For example, two processes—pregnancy, labor, and delivery and treatment for ischemic heart disease—accounted for 21 percent of care delivery costs at Intermountain. Leaders and staff then created crucial information systems around these key processes to track both clinical and financial data. They used these data to guide a restructuring of the organization that encouraged accountability and improvement that also relied on data.

Another strategy to improve processes and manage variation is skill building for staff. Some staff attend Intermountain's renowned Advanced Training Program (ATP), an intensive, twenty-day, year-long course for quality improvement leaders. ATP equips its participants with all the tools and competencies they will need to implement the kind of process management and improvement initiatives that Intermountain has been using to improve its care for decades. ATP is also a vital spread strategy, for this country and beyond, because executives and quality improvement leaders from all over attend the program and become members of a network of highly trained and committed improvers.

Intermountain found that a facility or system reorganized around key clinical processes ended up with a population health–driven business model. That financial incentives are still misaligned with this model continues to be an impediment, but leaders throughout health care are hoping that changes in payment structures beginning to take root will ease the way for reliable, evidence-based medicine to help drive down costs.

## Total Wellness: Southcentral Foundation

Attending to the health needs of native populations is a challenge for many western nations. The unique cultures and histories of native populations can be impediments to the successful application of western medicine. An organization in Anchorage, Alaska, has been addressing the needs of Alaska Natives since its incorporation thirty years ago and has emphasized a unique focus on the total wellness of this population. The Southcentral Foundation (SCF) currently manages both the Anchorage Native Primary Care Center and the Alaska Native Medical Center. Innovation has been at the heart of the organization's work since it began. The principal innovation SCF developed, and the one that guides all its work, is a system of care based on relationships. These key relationships—between providers and patients, patients and families, and families and communities—have transformed the quality of health care for the population served. The relationships are supported by full and open access to care, a focus on integration of mind and body, a commitment to measurement and quality, and a policy of giving power and control to the patient and family.

This special approach, which SCF calls the Nuka system of care (*nuka* is an Alaska Native word for strong, giant structures and living things), has resulted in dramatic and sustained improvements in hospital length of stay, use of emergency rooms and specialty services, health outcomes, and patient and staff satisfaction. Southcentral Foundation is continuously improving and innovating, developing new ways to improve care by improving relationships. By focusing on these relationships, SCF can improve the health of its patient population to a greater degree than traditional health care organizations focused solely on the patient-provider interaction can. In recent years, SCF has developed comprehensive workforce development programs, coaching and mentoring systems, and the Family Wellness Warriors initiative, which seeks to end domestic violence. All of SCF's work is grounded in the culture of Alaska Natives and all of it seeks to improve total wellness. Southcentral Foundation shows the power and potential of health care to improve health outside the walls of hospitals and clinics.

## Setting Aspirational Aims: Ascension Health

Ascension Health, the largest Catholic-owned health care system in the United States, understands the importance of setting aspirational goals. Unified under the promise of health care that works, health care that is safe, and health care that leaves no one behind, leaders at Ascension have set bold, some might say impossible goals for reducing errors and harm across their entire system. The Ascension Health initiative Getting to Zero, as its name suggests, sets goals that in many cases are zeroes: zero preventable deaths, zero preventable harm. When the system's project to eliminate birth trauma began, the national average was 6.59 instances of trauma per 1,000 live births. The Institute for Healthcare Improvement (IHI), one of Ascension's strategic partners, had set a goal for its birth trauma reduction initiative of 3.0 instances of trauma per 1,000 births. Ascension went further and set its goal at zero. Setting aspirational goals, especially goals like complete elimination, comes with the knowledge that failure is the likeliest result. But there is always learning in failure, and setting such lofty goals is motivating, even inspiring. And certainly failure is not the only result. Dozens and dozens of Ascension facilities met the goal of zero, completely eliminating birth trauma. Systemwide, the Getting to Zero push reduced pressure ulcers by 95 percent, neonatal mortality by 79 percent, birth trauma by 74 percent, ventilator-associated pneumonias by 56 percent, and falls with serious injuries by 54 percent. Doing what seems reasonable or possible can put us in what Paul Plsek (1997), engineer, author, and experienced advisor in quality improvement to complex organizations, calls mental valleys. Aiming for the (seemingly) impossible forces us to rethink assumptions, tear up old standards, and strive for perfection. Perfection achieved may be impossible, but the folks at Ascension Health learned that perfection pursued has tremendous value, and everyone should learn from that.

## Minimally Disruptive Medicine and Shared Decision Making: Mayo Health System

One of the beacons of high-quality, high-value health care in the United States is the Mayo Clinic Health System. Centered in Minnesota, Mayo also has facilities in Florida and Arizona. Mayo is famous around the world for groundbreaking clinical improvements, but it also has a strong and proud tradition in quality improvement. Two physicians working at the Mayo Clinic, Dr. Victor Montori and Dr. Henry Ting, have been looking at the way health care affects individuals. It's normal for clinicians to focus on the burden placed on the patient by her disease or condition. But what Montori and Ting are now looking at is the burden placed on the patient by the treatment of her condition. They want to develop what they call *minimally disruptive medicine.* It's a concept that requires coordination, communication, and engagement with patients and families.

The project is, in part, a response to the growing number of patients with multiple conditions. The complexity of caring for these conditions creates almost impossible situations for patients and families. Complex drug regimens and other treatments can easily overwhelm patients, resulting in patients skipping critical treatments in favor of less crucial ones owing to the difficulty of mentally managing all the moving parts. Take the example of medication treatments for diabetes. Drug regimens should be tailored to the specific situation and needs of the patient. For a condition like diabetes, there are many options and determining the right one is a difficult task that requires clinician engagement with the patient.

Ting and Montori, working through the Mayo Foundation for Medical Education and Research, developed medication cards to help ease this process. Each card lists the six most common diabetes medications and each card is labeled with a different criterion for selection. There's one that lists each drug's potential impact on lowering blood sugar, one that lays out the blood sugar monitoring required for each drug, one that lists side effects for each, one that explains the complexity of the daily routine, one that lists the possible impact on weight, and so on. The patient, in consultation with her caregiver, can determine which criteria are most important to her and which will have the most impact on her ability to adhere to the regimen. They then look at how each drug affects these criteria, and can select the regimen that fits her best. Standardization in medicine can be crucial, but tailoring treatment so it fits the patient is also essential. Americans are known for having busy lives, lives so busy that they negatively affect people's health. Making medicine less disruptive to people's lives and more customized to their needs and wishes can go a long way toward improving everyone's health.

## Using Lean Principles to Improve Care: Denver Health

With health care costs rising at unsustainable annual rates, health care organizations are increasingly turning to a well-tested method for reining in costs—lean thinking and production. The principles of lean, distilled from the Toyota Production System, are urgently needed in health care. Nearly all experts who look at health care costs in the United States agree about one thing— there is tremendous waste in the system. Duplicated tests, unnecessary procedures, byzantine record-keeping processes—all such activities drain the time and spirit of dedicated professionals. Applying lean principles and looking at value from the patient's perspective can help organizations see waste and drive it out of their systems. At Denver Health in Denver, Colorado, CEO Patricia Gabow has been using lean thinking since 2005. Gabow says, "We're getting good at getting better." She estimates that Denver Health has removed more than $100 million in waste as of 2011. Less money wasted on poorly designed administrative and clinical processes means more money for direct patient care. Eliminating health care waste can have a huge benefit for taxpayers too. In 2009, Denver Health's average length of stay for a Medicaid patient was shorter than the metro Denver average.

Medicaid charges from Denver Health were also more than 30 percent lower per day, and more than 35 percent lower per hospital stay, than the charges from the rest of Denver's facilities. Eliminating waste from health care is a necessary strategy to reduce costs and save entitlement programs. Denver Health and other health systems that use lean thinking (such as Virginia Mason Medical Center) are leading the way to lower costs and increased value.

## Collaborative Improvement
## QUEST: High Performing Hospitals

With innovation happening everywhere, harvesting the best ideas and spreading them throughout health care organizations everywhere is the next crucial step in fixing the U.S. health care system. For more than fifteen years, IHI has been running collaborative improvement projects in which groups of hospitals and other facilities join together to tackle specific problems while learning from and supporting each other. More recently, other organizations have taken up this method and are running large improvement projects targeting a wide variety of pressing issues. One of the largest and most successful of these initiatives is QUEST: High Performing Hospitals, a hospital collaborative project of Premier, Inc., a large alliance of hospitals and health care sites. QUEST's principles are familiar—to save lives; reduce costs; improve reliability, effectiveness, and safety; and improve the overall experience of patient care—but the initiative's scope and results are truly special. Comprising more than 200 hospitals across thirty-four states, QUEST is improving care and saving money on a large scale. The 157 charter member hospitals in the initiative have saved an estimated $2.85 billion in costs, and prevented the avoidable deaths of approximately 25,000 people. Measurement of and transparency about data are at the heart of QUEST. This focus on creating and using robust data systems is a model for all of health care. QUEST is also helping its participating facilities get ready for health care reform in the United States. As payments structures change and penalties for poor performance are introduced, QUEST participants will be uniquely prepared to thrive in the new environment.

## Building a New Kind of Medical School: Hofstra North Shore-LIJ School of Medicine

A growing and aging population is stressing the health care system in the United States. The rising number of patients with multiple conditions is making care more complex, with specialty care growing each year. The physician workforce is also aging. These and other reasons compelled the Association of American Medical Colleges to call for an increase in medical school enrollment of 30 percent by 2015. On top of this is an equally important need to refine the way physicians and nurses are educated in the United States. With complexity on the rise, and the near universal recognition that our health care workforce needs to be trained in the methods of improvement, there is a real need for innovation in medical education.

One of the first to take up this challenge is the Hofstra North Shore-LIJ School of Medicine at Hofstra University in Hempstead, New York. The new school will employ the combined resources and talents of Hofstra University and New York City's largest health system, North Shore-LIJ. The school, which convened its first class in the fall of 2011, will leverage advances in both medical and educational technology, becoming a model "millennial medical school." Innovation will be encouraged and incubated, and new techniques such as simulation will help students prepare for careers in twenty-first-century medicine. In addition to developing a new generation of physicians and other health professionals, the school is committed to changing and refining the way medicine is taught. Leaders at the school, at Hofstra, and at North Shore-LIJ also hope the school will look beyond academic medicine and have a measurable impact on the local community and improve the health of the population.

## Removing Barriers to Effective Care: NIATx

Treating patients with substance abuse or mental health problems is both extremely challenging for providers and extremely important to the U.S. health system. A group of innovators at the University of Wisconsin-Madison, led by Dave Gustafson, one of the founding members of IHI, have developed a simple, effective model for removing barriers to effective care and recovery for patients of providers and payers treating mental health problems or substance abuse.

The program is called NIATx (originally an acronym for Network for the Improvement of Addiction Treatment), and it is part of the University of Wisconsin Center for Health Enhancement Systems Studies (CHESS). It teaches a model that centers around four aims: reducing wait times between the initial request for treatment and the first session, reducing the number of no-shows, increasing admissions for treatment, and increasing the number of patients who continue treatment through at least four sessions. Each aim has its own metric and measurement strategy. The aims are supported by five core principles: understand and involve the customer, fix key problems, identify a charismatic and powerful change champion, find ideas for improvement from outside the field, and use rapid-cycle testing to demonstrate which changes are successful. From its original focus on addiction, NIATx has spread to mental health, and program leaders believe its approach can be applied to almost any part of the health system. The aims need to be adapted to the specific situation, but the core principles, as well as the identification and sharing of "promising practices" and the teaching of a collaborative learning system, are broadly spreadable. NIATx is a perfect example of how the science of improvement is being used to improve care in every corner of our health system.

## A Center for Innovation and Knowledge: Qulturum, Jönköping County

The idea of creating centers, within existing health care systems, devoted to learning, improvement, and innovation has been catching on in health care. The largest health system in New York City, North Shore-LIJ, operates a constantly growing and adapting Center for Learning and Innovation. One of the pioneers in this area works in a country with a national health system, a situation very different from that in the United States. Qulturum, an organization set up inside the health system of Jönköping County, Sweden, has been a leader in developing new ideas, testing them, and spreading them throughout the county and the entire country. Qulturum was established in 2000 and quickly created strong links to both the Institute for Healthcare Improvement and the Dartmouth Institute for Health Policy and Clinical Practice. Over the last ten years, Qulturum has helped Jönköping achieve some of the best clinical outcomes in Sweden, while keeping costs lower than most other counties' costs. Qulturum's strategy is to foster learning and innovation to achieve increased value for patients. It focuses on access and treating patients with respect and caring, prevention and self-care, cooperation and flow, clinical improvement, safety, and proper medication practices. One of the special things about Qulturum is its integration with both the health system and local government. By developing a genuine dialogue between the politicians that run the county and the clinical staff who run the hospitals, primary care centers, and specialty clinics, Qulturum has made quality improvement central to health care in the county. Through the persuasiveness of the county's results, and especially the generosity of its leaders and staff, the innovations developed in just one southern Swedish county are being spread throughout Sweden and into the rest of Europe as well. IHI is developing a Quality and Innovation Center (QIC) concept that is in many ways modeled on Qulturum. Delivering health care is a complex and weighty responsibility. It's difficult for overburdened staff and leaders—who are responsible to accreditors and in some cases also to stockholders as well as to patients—to find the time and resources to devote to innovation and learning. Qulturum is an ideal model for the kind of organization needed in health care systems if care is going to be transformed in the ways it needs to be.

## The Productive Series: NHS Institute for Innovation and Improvement

Sweden is not the only country in Europe breaking new ground on quality improvement. In England the National Health Service (NHS England) is charged with providing care to more than fifty million people, making it the largest single-payer health system in the world. Improving efficiency, quality, and safety is of special importance to such an enormous system. The organization responsible for these improvements is the NHS Institute for Innovation and Improvement. The Institute has in recent years developed a series of tools and case studies that empower staff to effect real change for the facilities they work in. It is called the Productive Series. Like so many other improvement initiatives, the Productive Series relies on efficiency improvement methods that originated in manufacturing and safety improvements first developed in aviation. The Productive Series aims to transform the culture of health care to one of safety and continuous improvement. So far, the institute has created seven different series, for facilities ranging from office practices to mental health facilities. When England began instituting fiscal austerity measures, resulting in unprecedented budget cuts to the NHS, these tools for improving care while reducing costs became even more important. They also hold real value for health care leaders outside England as well because so many of the concepts used are simple and broadly applicable.

## Changing a Whole Country: Patient Safety Programs in Scotland and Denmark

One of the reasons we wrote this book was to argue that if the innovations presented here could be spread across this entire country, the United States would be well on its way out of its health care crisis. Other nations face similar crises and in some instances have instituted national programs mandating the spread of proven, evidence-based practices to make care safer and better. An advantage of being a smaller country with a highly integrated health system is the ability to rally that system around a single goal and move toward national improvement. No country has demonstrated this will to improve at a national level more than Scotland. Working within NHS Scotland, Healthcare Improvement Scotland partnered with IHI to design the Scottish Patient Safety Programme (SPSP). This program, which focuses on leadership, critical (intensive) care, general ward (medical-surgical) care, medicines management, and postoperative care, is being implemented in every acute care hospital in Scotland. Program leaders plan to spread the program to pediatrics and primary care services in the coming years. The program relies on several primary drivers of success, including the Scottish government setting patient safety as a strategic priority, local and national boards setting safety as a priority, building a sustainable infrastructure for improvement, and aligning with existing national improvement goals and measures. By carefully tending to these key strategies, the program has begun to transform safety in Scottish hospitals, saving lives and averting countless instances of needless harm.

A slightly different model is being applied in Denmark, as part of the Danish Safer Hospital Program. The Danish Society for Patient Safety and representatives from the Danish regions are partnering to make care dramatically safer for all patients in Denmark. Starting small, the program is beginning with five hospitals in various regions across Denmark, and is focusing on the same areas as those targeted in Scotland (leadership, critical care, general ward care, medicines management, and postoperative care). The results achieved in the initiative will be broadly shared and disseminated as an inspiration to the rest of the nation's health care system.

National initiatives to improve care in the United States are not unprecedented. IHI's 100,000 and 5 Million Lives campaigns engaged over four thousand hospitals, representing more than 80 percent of U.S. hospital beds. Still, it's hard to imagine a national program like the one in Scotland being implemented in every U.S. hospital. However, individual states are trying this approach. In South Carolina, the South Carolina Hospital Association is leading a program called Safe Surgery 2015: South Carolina, through which all sixty-one acute care hospitals in the state will implement the World Health Organization's surgical safety checklist. This is just one of many examples of state hospital associations running large-scale initiatives. And regions smaller than states can also be organized to collaborate toward improved care, as the city of Memphis has done by creating a coalition to engage in IHI's Triple Aim in a Region initiative.

# References

August, J. (2010, November 22). A blueprint for whole systems improvement. *LMPtalk* [Blog]. Retrieved November 11, 2011, from http://www.lmpartnership.org/lmptalk/blogs/history-future/blueprint-whole-systems-improvement.

Berwick, D. M., Nolan, T. W., & Whittington, J. (2008, May/June). The Triple Aim: Care, health, and cost. *Health Affairs*, pp. 759–769.

Blackmore, C. C., Mecklenburg, R. S., & Kaplan, G. S. (2011). Effectiveness of clinical decision support in controlling inappropriate imaging. *Journal of the American College of Radiology, 8*(1), 19–25.

Blue Cross Blue Shield of Massachusetts. (2011, July 14). *Harvard Medical School researchers find Alternative Quality Contract lowers spending and improves patient care* [News release]. Boston: Author. Retrieved November 1, 2011, from http://www.bluecrossma.com/visitor/newsroom/press-releases/2011/newsRelease07142011.html.

Christensen, C. (1997). *The innovator's dilemma: When new technologies cause great firms to fail.* Boston: Harvard Business Review Press.

Commonwealth Fund. (2010a, June/July). A conversation with Dana Gelb Safran about getting the incentives right: The Blue Cross Blue Shield of Massachusetts Alternative Quality Contract. *Quality Matters.* Retrieved November 2, 2011, from http://www.commonwealthfund.org/Content/Newsletters/Quality-Matters/2010/June-July-2010/A-Conversation-with-Dana-Safran.aspx.

Commonwealth Fund. (2010b, June/July). Case study: The Mount Auburn Cambridge Independent Practice Association. *Quality Matters.* Retrieved November 2, 2011, from http://www.commonwealthfund.org/Newsletters/Quality-Matters/2010/June-July-2010/Case-Study.aspx.

Convergence Partnership. (2010, May 28). Letter to US Department of Health and Human Services Secretary Kathleen Sibelius. Retrieved

January 30, 2012, from http://www.convergencepartnership.org/atf/cf/%7B245a9b44-6ded-4abd-a392-ae583809e350%7D/CP%20-%20CEO%20LETTER%20PREVENTION%20FUND.PDF

DiGioia, A., 3rd., Greenhouse, P. K., & Levison, T. J. (2007, October). Patient and family-centered collaborative care: An orthopaedic model. *Clinical Orthopaedics and Related Research, 463*, 13–19.

Dudl, R.J., Wang, M.C., Wong, M., & Bellows, J. (2009, October 1). Preventing myocardial infarction and stroke with a simplified bundle of cardioprotective medications. *American Journal of Managed Care*, pp. e88-e94.

Fox, S.; Blue Cross Blue Shield of Massachusetts. (2011, May 13). *Changing the way we pay for care: The move to global payments.* Presentation at the Massachusetts League of Community Health Centers annual conference. Retrieved November 3, 2011, from http://www.massleague.org/Calendar/LeagueEvents/CHI/2011/MAMarketplace.pdf.

Gawande, A. (2011, May 26). Cowboys and pit crews. *New Yorker* Web site. Retrieved December 9, 2011, from http://www.newyorker.com/online/blogs/newsdesk/2011/05/atul-gawande-harvard-medical-school-commencement-address.html.

Guterman, S., Schoenbaum, S. C., Davis, K., Schoen, C., Audet, A.-M.J., Stremikis, K., et al. (2011). *High performance accountable care: Building on success and learning from experience.* Washington, DC: Commonwealth Fund.

Health Care Incentives Improvement Institute. (2011). *What is Prometheus Payment?* Retrieved November 2, 2011, from http://www.hci3.org/what_is_prometheus.

HealthPartners. (2011). *Optimal diabetes care* [Fact sheet]. Retrieved October 20, 2011, from http://www.healthpartners.com/public/about/triple-aim/optimal-diabetes-care.

Herzlinger, R. E. (1997). *Market-driven health care: Who wins, who loses in the transformation of America's largest service industry.* New York: Basic Books.

Hostetter, M. (2011, April/May). Case study: Legacy Clinic Emanuel—Increasing access and efficiency through team-based primary care. *Quality Matters.* Retrieved October 30, 2011, from http://www.commonwealthfund.org/Newsletters/Quality-Matters/2011/April-May-2011/Case-Study.aspx.

Improving Chronic Illness Care, Group Health Research Institute. (1998). *The chronic care model.* Retrieved October 20, 2011, from http://www.improvingchroniccare.org/index.php?p=The_Chronic_Care_Model&s=2.

Institute for Clinical Systems Improvement. (2010). *ICSI 2010 annual report: Targeting the Triple Aim.* Bloomington, MN: Author.

Institute for Healthcare Improvement. (2003). *The Breakthrough Series: IHI's collaborative model for achieving breakthrough improvement* (IHI Innovation Series white paper). Boston: Author.

Institute of Medicine, Committee on Quality of Health Care in America. (2001). *Crossing the quality chasm: A new health system for the 21st century.* Washington, DC: National Academies Press.

Institute of Medicine Roundtable on Value and Science-Driven Health Care. *Member Spotlight: George Halvorson, Kaiser Permanente.* Retrieved January 30, 2012, from http://www.iom.edu/Activities/Quality/VSRT/~/media/Files/Activity%20Files/Quality/VSRT/Spotlights/KP.pdf.

Intel Corporation. (n.d.[a]). *Intel supplier quality portal.* Retrieved October 27, 2011, from https://supplier.intel.com/static/Quality.

Intel Corporation. (n.d.[b]). Moore's law and Intel innovation. *About Intel.* Retrieved October 27, 2011, from http://www.intel.com/about/companyinfo/museum/exhibits/moore.htm.

Isham, G. (2011, March/April). Minnesota and the emerging ACO. *MetroDoctors* (The Journal of the Twin Cities Medical Society), pp. 23–25.

Kaiser Permanente. (2005, July 6). *"Thrive" ad campaign changing consumer perceptions of Kaiser Permanente* [News release]. Retrieved November 13, 2011, from http://ckp.kp.org/newsroom/national/archive/nat_050722_newthrive.html.

Klein, S., & McCarthy, D. (2010, July). *CareOregon: Transforming the role of a Medicaid health plan from payer to partner.* Washington, DC: Commonwealth Fund.

Kohn, L. T., Corrigan, J. M., & Donaldson, M. S. (Eds.); Committee on Quality of Health Care in America, Institute of Medicine. (2000). *To err is human: Building a safer health system.* Washington, DC: National Academies Press.

Kotter, J. (1996). *Leading change.* Boston: Harvard Business Press.

Labby, D., Read, D., & Winkel, A. (2011, February). *Towards a new model of primary care: Early results from the Primary Care Renewal initiative: Decreased cost, better care, better patient experience.* Retrieved October 31, 2011, from http://www.communityclinics.org/section/library/?topic=1&subtopics=11&page=3.

Langley, G.J., Moen, R., Nolan, K.M., Nolan, T.W., Norman, C.L., Provost, L.P. (2009). *The improvement guide: A practical approach to enhancing organizational performance, 2nd Edition.* San Francisco: Jossey-Bass.

Levy, P. (2011, March 17). The Inspector General observes. *Not Running a Hospital* [Blog]. Retrieved November 3, 2011, from http://runningahospital.blogspot.com/2011/03/inspector-general-observes.html.

Liebermann, J. R. (2010, May). How to build a culture of innovation from the inside out. *The Health Care Blog* [Blog]. Retrieved November 13, 2011, from http://thehealthcareblog.com/blog/2010/05/21/how-to-build-a-culture-of-innovation-from-the-inside-out.

Lorber, D. (2011, July). *Health care spending and quality in year 1 of the Alternative Quality Contract* (In the Literature series). Washington, DC: Commonwealth Fund.

Massoud, M. R., Nielsen, G. A., Nolan, K., Schall, M. W., & Sevin, C. (2006). *A framework for spread: From local improvements to system-wide change* (IHI Innovation Series white paper). Cambridge, MA: Institute for Healthcare Improvement. Retrieved November 11, 2011, from http://www.ihi.org/knowledge/Pages/IHIWhitePapers/AFrameworkforSpreadWhitePaper.aspx.

Merchant, N. (2011, March 22). Culture trumps strategy, every time. HBR Blog Network. Retrieved December 9, 2011, from http://blogs.hbr.org/cs/2011/03/culture_trumps_strategy_every.html.

Meyer, G., Nelson, E., Pryor, D., James, B., Swensen, S., Kaplan, G., et al. (In press). More quality measures vs. measuring what matters: A call for balance and parsimony. *New England Journal of Medicine.*

Meyer, H. (2011). At UPMC, improving care processes to serve patients better and cut costs. *Health Affairs, 30*(3), 400–403.

Minnesota Community Measurement. (2010). *2010 Health care disparities report for Minnesota health care programs.* Minneapolis, MN: Author.

Nichols, L. M. (2010). Perspective: Be not afraid. *New England Journal of Medicine, 362*, e30.

Nolan, T. (2007). *Execution of strategic improvement initiatives to produce system-level results* (IHI Innovation Series white paper). Cambridge, MA: Institute for Healthcare Improvement.

Nolan, T., Nolan, K., Henderson, S., & Lynn, J. (2010, October) *IHI 90-day R&D project final report: Triple Aim in a region, Part 2.* Cambridge, MA: Institute for Healthcare Improvement.

NuVal. (2011). How it works. *NuVal.* Retrieved November 5, 2011, from http://www.nuval.com/How.

PFCC Partners of UPMC. (2008). *PFCC business story: A methodology to building high performance teams.* Pittsburgh, PA: The Innovation Center of UPMC. Retrieved November 9, 2011, from http://innovationctr.org/resources.

Plsek, P. P. (1997). *Creativity, innovation, and quality.* Milwaukee, WI: ASQ Quality Press.

Porter, M. E., & Teisberg, E. O. (2006). *Redefining health care.* Boston: Harvard Business Review Press.

Porter, M. E., Teisberg, E. O., & Wallace, S. (2008, July 16). What should employers do about health care? *HBS Working Knowledge* [E-mail newsletter]. Retrieved November 1, 2011, from http://hbswk.hbs.edu/item/5979.html.

Pugh, M., & Reinertsen, J. (2007, November/December). Reducing harm to patients. *Healthcare Executive.* Retrieved November 11, 2011, from http://findarticles.com/p/articles/mi_hb5693/is_200711/ai_n32244826.

Reinertsen, J. (2003). Zen and the art of physician autonomy maintenance. *Annals of Internal Medicine, 138*(12), 992–995.

Robert Wood Johnson Foundation. (2011). *What is Prometheus Payment? An evidence-informed model for payment reform.* Retrieved December 8, 2011, from http://www.rwjf.org/files/research/prometheusmodeljune09.pdf

Schoen, C., Osborn, R., Doty, M. M., Bishop, M., Peugh, J., & Murukutla, N. (2007). Toward higher-performance health systems: Adults' health care experiences in seven countries. *Health Affairs* [Web Exclusive], *26*(6), w717–w734.

Schoen, C., Osborn, R., Squires, D., Doty, M., Pierson, R., Applebaum, S. (2011). New 2011 survey of patients with complex care needs in eleven countries finds that care is often poorly coordinated. *Health Affairs, 30*(12), w2437–w2448.

Schroeder, S. A. (2007). We can do better—Improving the health of the American people. *New England Journal of Medicine, 357,* 1221–1228.

Song, Z., Safran, D. G., Landon, B. E., He, Y., Ellis, R. P., Mechanic, R. E., et al. (2011). Health care spending and quality in year 1 of the Alternative Quality Contract. *New England Journal of Medicine, 365,* 909–918.

Sperl-Hillen, J. M., Averbeck, B., Palattao, K., Amundson, J., Ekstrom, H., MA, Rush, B., et al. (2010). Outpatient EHR-based diabetes clinical decision support that works: Lessons learned from implementing Diabetes Wizard. *Diabetes Spectrum, 23*(3), 150–154. Retrieved October 20, 2011, from http://spectrum.diabetesjournals.org/content/23/3/150.full.

Steenhuysen, J. (2009, October 1). Cheap three-drug combination helps cut heart risks. Reuters. Retrieved January 30, 2012, from http://www.reuters.com/article/2009/10/01/us-heart-drugs-idUSTRE5907LR20091001.

Wallace, P. (Spring 2005). The Care Management Institute: Making the right thing easier to do. *The Permanente Journal,* pp. 56–57. http://www.ncbi.nlm.nih.gov/pubmed/21660163

# Index